THE MOTHERHOOD DIET

For Miraculous Babies

Author

Hakan COKSUER, MD., Assoc. Prof.

Translated by
Yasemin Unlusoy

Editorial Consultant
Mursel Cavus

Publisher

Cosmo Publishing Company

ISBN: 978-1-949872-06-4

PREFACE **1**

CHAPTER 1 .... **5**

FERTILITY, THE FRUITFULNESS OF THE HUMAN BODY *7*

CHAPTER 2 .... **19**

FERTILITY SYMPTOMS *21*
GETTING READY FOR PREGNANCY *27*
IDEAL WEIGHT CALCULATOR BASED ON AGE AND HEIGHT ... *34*
PSYCHOLOGICAL AND MENTAL READINESS FOR THE DIET *37*

CHAPTER 3 .... **43**

PRE-CONCEPTION NUTRITION *45*
FOOD GROUPS *51*
THE EFFECTS OF BEVERAGES ON FERTILITY *74*
FERTILITY ENHANCING FOODS *80*
NUTRITION ON SPECIAL DAYS *85*
HOW TO DO A FERTILITY DETOX *87*
FERTILITY MASSAGE *94*
SAMPLE DIET THAT WILL INCREASE YOUR FERTILITY *97*
7-DAY FALL MENU *99*
7-DAY WINTER MENU *106*
7-DAY SPRING MENU *113*
7-DAY SUMMER MENU *120*
MALE FACTOR & MALE FERTILITY *129*

CHAPTER 5 .... **139**

DISEASES AND NUTRITION *141*
THE MOST COMMON MYTHS ABOUT FERTILITY *147*

CHAPTER 6 .... **151**

FREQUENTLY ASKED QUESTIONS *153*
SOURCES: *163*

***The dietary suggestions in this book were developed in cooperation with a dietitian.**

PREFACE

"The relationship between fertility and nutrition is far stronger than our expectations," Md. Coksuer said in our first meeting. "I advise my patients to eat healthy even before we start the in vitro fertilization treatment. There have been many cases where women were able to become pregnant by eating more healthfully. Therefore, books and recipes focusing on that issue are always needed."

I realized that Coksuer was emphasizing the importance of studying a subject in depth, and that was something we had in common. He was knowledgeable and well educated. After graduating from Trakya University in 2001, he specialized in obstetrics and gynecology at Zeynep Kamil Training and Research Hospital, the most highly regarded medical institution for obstetrics and gynecology in Turkey. From pelvic reconstruction to aesthetic gynecology, molecular biology and genetics to andrology, laparoscopy and in vitro fertilization, he had worked in numerous fields. Having published articles on infertility in many scientific publications, Coksuer was not only employing Western medicine but also Eastern medicine, and he had training in acupuncture as well. For Coksuer, it's vital to care for health holistically, beyond just treating symptoms. "This book is designed to increase the fertility of mothers, and I even have a goal beyond that," he says. "I want to have a role in the birth of healthier babies. In order for all of us to welcome healthier babies, future mothers have to start their fertility nutrition at least three months before pregnancy."

Associate Professor Hakan Coksuer's first book ***The Motherhood Diet for Miraculous Babies*** included some background information on how mothers should prepare their bodies for pregnancy, as well as some weekly sample menus showing what should be eaten during different seasons. Was that enough? Of course not! The pregnancy diet is not just about eating the recommended food. Every detail is important to consider, from the right choice of vegetables and fruits to the selection of the cookware, cooking techniques, and dealing with the risk of contamination. Therefore, we had to create new recipes. In ***Fertility Cookbook*** *for Perfect Babies*, this is exactly what Coksuer does. The recipes, including nutrition that best supports fertility, are carefully prepared based on the best cooking techniques and other details. Under the supervision of a nutritionist, selected ingredients were transformed into recipes by a recipe writing specialist. They were cooked, tasted and revised continually. To have our photo shoot featuring natural fruits and vegetables fresh in season, we even had to wait for the right season to come. That is why it took years to prepare this book.

For all these reasons, you can be assured that you can cook these recipes with contentment and enjoy delicious food while feeling confident that you'll not only increase your fertility but also do your best for your baby's health.

Mursel Cavus

İstanbul, 2017

Hakan Coksuer MD, Assoc. Prof.

He was born in Mardin in 1977. He completed his high school education in Istanbul.

In 2001, he graduated from Trakya University and received the title of Medical Doctor.

In 2006, he became a Gynecologist and Obstetrician in Istanbul Zeynep Kamil Training and Research Hospital and received pelvic reconstruction surgery training at the same hospital.

He started his master's degree program in Molecular Biology and Genetics in Istanbul.

In 2008, he started to work as an assistant professor at Dumlupınar University. He worked in Ankara GATA Obstetrics and Gynecology Department between 2010 and 2011 and completed his education about "tube baby" there.

He received a master's degree in the field of Health Institutions Management at Ankara Turkish Air Institution University.

Between 2010 and 2013, he was the president of the Turkish Society of Gynecology and Obstetrics in Kütahya (TJOD). In 2012, during he received the second prize for Polycystic Ovarian Syndrome during TJOD Congress.

He completed medical ozone therapy training. He is a referee in the field of infertility and gynecology in the magazines such as Archives of Gynecology and Obstetrics,

Gynecology and Obstetrics and Gynecological Endocrinology which are the most respected magazines of European.

He completed his doctoral program in clinical psychology. Coksuer, which also has Laparoscopy and Acupuncture certificates, has published 34 domestic and 30 overseas articles.

Hıs first book is "Stresi Akupunktur ile Yendim Tüp Bebeğe Hazırım”. Coksuer speaks Turkish and English.

Chapter One

FERTILITY,

THE FRUITFULNESS OF THE HUMAN BODY

Most people think getting pregnant is a walk in the park. Yet, once the decision is made to have a baby, many couples discover it is not that easy. In simple terms, fertility can be defined as a woman's ability to fall pregnant and a man's ability to impregnate. Infertility, on the other hand, is the failure to achieve a pregnancy for both sexes as a result of sexual intercourse. Of course, absence of pregnancy during the first few months of trial does not mean infertility. According to the definition of World Health Organization, infertility comes to the fore when a couple cannot conceive a child after at least twelve months of regular unprotected sexual intercourse.

As a physician, I have concentrated on in vitro fertilization for years. During this process, I recognized that the factors causing infertility are not limited to health issues. Other determinants play a role, such as dietary habits, the couple's psychological state, rest, hormonal balances, age, weight, lifestyle, stress level, current medications, smoking and drinking.

You may consider the book you are holding in your hands, which I wrote in light of this fact, as a guide for your pregnancy preparation process. **The Motherhood Diet for Miraculous Babies** aims not only to give you nutritional advice but also to explain how female fertility functions and to share with you the information you need regarding a healthier diet for you and your baby. If you live in harmony with your own nature and can manage yourself in this sense, you will discover that your body was created to generate another life in this world

Let's first consider the factors that affect the conception process and female fertility, as we focus on the fertility of prospective mothers in this book.

The Process of Conception

Quite complex and fragile processes are at work in a prospective mother's body during pre-conception and conception. As the saying goes, "two cells and a miracle are necessary to generate a life." That miracle is created by very delicate hormonal balances and physiological changes in a woman's body. A complex, collaborative and triggering system goes into operation, where secretions of hormones in certain parts of the brain, certain transmitters in the blood, hormone-producing organs in the abdomen, and the reactions of other organs to such stimuli are all orchestrated.

We all know that egg and sperm cells must unite to start a pregnancy. However, there is more to it earlier on. A 'healthy' sperm cell is needed from the prospective father, just like a healthy egg is needed from the prospective mother's body. Women have two ovaries, one on the right and one on the left. There is a multitude of follicles that are waiting to mature in each ovary. Ovaries are stimulated by the hormones to mature an egg and release it into the fallopian tube every 28 days. Occasionally, twin and triplet pregnancies can occur if multiple eggs are matured and sent into the fallopian tubes with the impact of hormones. The mature egg in the fallopian tube constitutes the first cell of a baby by uniting with the sperm that comes from the prospective father. The genetic codes of mother and father unite, and the first stage of a process that is essential for the formation of a brand-new life is completed. The new cell sets off on its journey to a suitable and protective spot in the womb while self-dividing simultaneously, and proceeds with its segmentation after it implants in the uterus. Over the course of the next nine months, that one cell transforms into billions of cells, creating a tiny human being.

In other words, the first phase of fertility requires ovaries to mature a healthy egg and release it into the fallopian tube prior to the union of two cells, and this process must be orchestrated by a balanced hormonal system.

Hormones

The key players that affect the health of ovulation and sperm production are hormones and their transmitters. Let's look at the hormones and transmitters that are important to us in order to better understand the impact of diet on fertility.

GnRH, FSH and LH: GnRH (gonadotropin-releasing hormone) secreted by the hypothalamus in the brain stimulates the pituitary gland and regulates the secretions of **FSH** (follicle stimulating hormon) and **LH** (luteinizing hormone). These two hormones undertake the key task in the regulation of reproduction. While FSH stimulates the growth and maturation of ova (egg cells), LH helps these ova crack and be released into the fallopian tubes.

Estrogen: Estrogen, the key player in the female reproductive system, is released by the follicles (the structure that encapsulates and protects the egg cell) and, once again, the secretion of this hormone depends on FSH. Estrogen prepares a protective bed for the implantation and growth of the self-dividing cell coming down the fallopian tube by enabling the development and thickening of the endometrium (inner lining of womb), which is important for the fertilized egg to attach itself to the womb.

Progesterone: Progesterone, which also affects the ovulation cycle, is produced by corpus luteum (yellow substance released when the follicle ruptures during ovulation) under the supervision of LH, and it helps estrogen with the development of the womb's inner lining.

Carrier Globulin [1] : These are the carriers that accompany hormones by getting attached to them, because tissues outside of the related systems will also be affected when hormones hang around in the blood by themselves. Globulin, which is the carrier of sex hormones, prevents an unwanted impact on untargeted tissues by enabling a balanced and regulated circulation of hormones. Estrogen and testosterone are present in both males and females. Of course, estrogen levels in females are vastly higher than in males, while testosterone in males far outweighs testosterone in females. Due to its structure, globulin likes attaching itself to testosterone more than to estrogen. Therefore, a low level of globulin translates into the free roaming of the male hormone testosterone in a female's blood vessels and tissues at a higher level. Medically, this is not desirable. Globulin prevents negative impacts on fertility by inhibiting a rise in testosterone level in a woman's body. Accordingly, not only the levels of hormones but also the levels of carriers play a considerable role in pregnancy.

Insulin: Insulin is a critical hormone, for it is directly affected by our dietary habits and affects plenty of systems

---

[1] **Globulin:** One of the substances in blood plasma, a protein of large molecules.

as well as fertility. It is produced in the pancreas, and its main role is the regulation of blood sugar.

If there is continuous insulin secretion and above-normal insulin levels in the bloodstream, cells perceive insulin as a growth hormone, because insulin and growth factor structures are very similar to each other. This overstimulation causes the cells to act in a marginal manner and change their activities. This, in turn, leads to a growth in the cells. At the same time, insulin affects sex hormones such as estrogen and testosterone, which regulate reproduction.

A well-balanced blood sugar level throughout the day is important in terms of health and fertility. To balance blood sugar through diet, an individual need to have regular meals, following a program of six meals/snacks per day, emphasizing grains and dark wheat, legumes, fruits with lower sugar content, dairy products as a second food group and low-calorie food that is not labelled as "light."

To a great extent, the Motherhood Diet is built on proper management of blood sugar. Spiking blood sugar levels increase insulin resistance and the risk of developing type 2 diabetes. Sudden increases in blood sugar stimulate the pancreas continuously and trigger insulin secretion. Elevated insulin levels repress the function of globulin, and globulin cannot control the male testosterone hormone sufficiently in the blood. A high level of testosterone that roams free in the blood may cause unwanted effects on female reproductive health. Elevated levels of insulin and testosterone can also lead to ovarian cysts that inhibit ovulation, a disease called polycystic ovary syndrome (PCOS).

It is surprising to see how the sugar type and content of our food choices can affect ovulation even though, in theory, they may not have any harmful or toxic effects. It will be helpful to keep this in mind while analyzing the potential effects of your food choices on your body.

Leptin: Leptin, one of the hormones that is secreted by fat cells and affects reproduction, is important in many respects, including weight control. Fat cells send the message of "I am full" by secreting this hormone after storing fat and becoming enlarged, in other words after absorbing enough. On the other hand, leptin secretion decreases when the body is truly hungry. Studies of this hormone, which was discovered by Homolog Yiying Zhang, indicate certain impacts on the reproductive system after prolonged fasting results in lower levels of leptin. Ovulation in women and sperm production in men decline after prolonged fasting. If you eat regularly and do not stay hungry for very long, these negative effects will disappear.

Thyroid: Thyroxine (T4), triiodothyronine (T3), and calcitonin, produced and secreted by the thyroid gland, are called thyroid hormones. The thyroid gland, located right below the Adam's apple in the throat, is actually an endocrine gland, and metabolism is regulated by these hormones to a substantial extent. In a sense, the thyroid gland is like an orchestra conductor in the body, directing many functions, ranging from heart rate to cholesterol level and from memory to skin structure.

The levels of thyroid hormones in the blood are regulated by a hormone that stimulates the TSH-thyroid gland. TSH is secreted when thyroid hormones decrease in the bloodstream, and conversely, TSH secretion decreases when thyroid hormones increase. An overactive or underactive thyroid gland causes irregular menstrual cycles as well as an increase in the amount of menstrual bleeding. This, in turn, seriously affects female fertility. Thyroid hormones should always be within the normal range, because this type of hormonal disorder can affect the outcome of pregnancy endeavors or IVF treatment. It can also give rise to undesirable effects on the mother and baby during pregnancy. Therefore, diagnosis and treatment of thyroid issues are important.

Thyroid gland disorders can develop before or during pregnancy. Symptoms of thyroid disease such as vomiting, nausea, exhaustion, palpitation, and lack of appetite may be confused with pregnancy symptoms, and this can delay its diagnosis and treatment. Attention should be paid to this in early pregnancy, a period during which pregnancy hormones reach their maximum values.

In summary, the delicate balance of hormones confronts us with an important argument in terms of the pre-pregnancy and pregnancy stages. In this book, we will be discussing the impact of our dietary habits on hormones that sustain and strengthen fertility and the ways we can keep this balance through diet.

Physical Health

A number of physical conditions may also hinder pregnancy, other than hormones affected by our lifestyle and dietary habits. Consult your doctor right away when you decide to get pregnant, to see whether a condition is affecting your health.

Nearly 10% of women are affected by PCOS. Many tiny cysts are observed on the ovarian walls of women who suffer from PCOS, and these cysts can hinder oogenesis (egg development). We previously mentioned that a rise in insulin and testosterone increases the probability of PCOS. It is obvious that even this disease, which physically impedes us, is related to healthy eating and dietary habits.

Certain cervical conditions can prevent the sperm from entering the uterus and fertilizing the egg. Similarly, polyps in the uterus can interfere with the implantation of the fertilized egg on the inner lining. A cohesion, tightness, or any kind of physical problem in the fallopian tubes, where sperm and egg meet, can also hinder pregnancy by creating an obstacle for fertilization. Tests should be conducted to rule out any vaginal infections as well. Studies show that 15% of infertility cases stem from vaginal infections.

However, do not give in to despair by thinking that the aforementioned conditions will prevent pregnancy. You need to trust your body's strength and the inner hope for motherhood that is inherent in your nature, in addition to small medical procedures and medications.

Ovarian Reserve

The ovarian reserve refers to the quantity, quality and state of the eggs that are present in the ovaries of a woman. In other words, it refers to a woman's capacity to get pregnant. Each female is born with a certain number of eggs, and the number of healthy eggs diminishes as years go by. While the pregnancy outcome probability for a healthy 30-year-old woman is around 20%, ovarian reserve decreases as she gets older, especially after the age of 35. Chance of pregnancy decreases, and the risk of miscarriage increases for a woman with diminished ovarian capacity. I highly recommend that you have your ovarian reserve measured if you are planning for pregnancy currently or in the future.

The factors leading to a decrease in ovarian reserve can be specified as age, excessive weight, smoking, certain ovarian operations, endometriosis [2], chemotherapy and radiotherapy exposure.

Age

The impact of age on fertility is indisputable. The physiological changes that occur over time lead to a decrease in cervical fluid and frequency of ovulation. While the risk of miscarriage increases directly proportional with age, it is also possible to get pregnant and have a healthy pregnancy at later ages. You can partially forestall the impact of aging on fertility by changing your life and dietary habits.

Stress

Physical and mental stress can delay or even stop ovulation. Yet, I also have some good news for you. An eight-year stress study conducted in the USA on over 30,000 adults revealed that if you think stress is bad for you and affects you negatively, your risk of premature death rises to 43%; and if you think stress keeps you dynamic, this risk goes down to almost 0. This shows the extent the mind can be influential on the body and the health of a human being. For this reason, refrain from thinking of stress as a bad thing. Should you want further information on this, I highly recommend you watch Kelly McGonigal's video of "How to make stress your friend" on www.ted.com

---

[2] **Endometriosis:** A disorder in which the inner tissue, or the inner lining of uterus that is shed during menstruation, grows outside of the uterus.

However, do not overlook the fact that excessive stress alters the hormonal balance in the body, while a certain dose of it keeps the body dynamic. Accordingly, you need to carefully observe yourself and your body's reaction to stress. Is stress motivating you, or is it affecting you adversely? You need to learn how to manage your stress while taking your own personality into account.

Toxins

It is not possible to completely get rid of the toxins that surround us all in our daily lives. According to research, at present our bodies are exposed to about 30,000–50,000 chemical substances that our grandparents were never exposed to. This, in turn, leads to escalation of many diseases. Genital birth defects have increased by four times in Europe. We get our share of toxins from pesticides, the biggest contaminators of surface and ground water, and this damages hormonal balance. To reduce the effects of chemicals, it's important to eliminate alcohol and smoking, cosmetics with chemical content, and chemical cleaning agents from our lives as much as possible, while consciously choosing fresh and organic food and hygiene products.

A toxic load or toxic burden arises because of excessive accumulation of toxins in your body. Please have a look at the following symptoms and note the ones you experience in the table to see whether you might have such a toxic burden.

TOXIC LOAD TABLE	
1	*Fatigue and sleepiness, especially after meals*
2	*Increasing loss of concentration*
3	*Waking up tired in the morning*
4	*Gas, bloating, nausea, bellyache*
5	*Constipation*
6	*Weight gain*
7	*Cranky joints and bones*
8	*Frequent upper respiratory and urinary tract problems*
9	*Kidney and gallstones*
10	*Fatty liver*
11	*Hypertension*
12	*Fluctuations and upsurges in fasting blood glucose*

Nutrition

I have already mentioned that diet and reproduction are far more related than we think. Hormone levels and the way hormones function are affected by our dietary habits. Nutrition is a complex and comprehensive process. After you get a bite of something, miscellaneous factors are at play, ranging from the interaction of food with saliva enzymes, to digestive functions of stomach, to the ensuing process in the intestines—the longest organ in your body—to the method of cooking used, the amount consumed, the interaction of different food items eaten together, and even the way an item travels to your plate from the farm. All of these affect the way food is used by your body. Endeavoring to follow the dietary suggestions presented in this book is crucial to preparing your body for a healthy pregnancy and looking forward to a healthy and joyful encounter with the little one who will develop and grow in your womb over the course of forty weeks.

The dietary style I will provide you with has been designed to boost the pregnancy rate. For this reason, I encourage you to start following it at least six months prior to the initiation of your pregnancy attempts. Taking the vitamins and other supplements prescribed by your physician during regular checkups is also highly important for you and your future baby's health.

Chapter Two

FERTILITY SYMPTOMS

The fertility window of a prospective mother depends on her menstrual cycle. This cycle is usually 28 days and can vary for each woman. If you know the ovulation period within your menstrual cycle, you can predict the time you will be most prone to getting pregnant. Let's have a look at the phases of the menstrual cycle and the period in which you have the highest chance for conception.

In the menstrual cycle, the period up until ovulation is called the "follicular phase," because follicles are developing in the ovaries, or the "proliferative phase" due to the thickening of endometrium. The period after ovulation, on the other hand, is called the "luteal" or "secretory" phase.

Follicular Phase

During this period, which starts on the first day of menstruation, the brain starts secreting the previously mentioned FSH hormone to enable the maturation of an egg in the ovaries. As the egg grows and matures, it secretes estrogen and prepares the lining of the uterus for pregnancy. Within just a few weeks, the LH secreted by the pituitary gland causes the egg to be released. The progesterone secreted by the corpus luteum (yellow body) causes the body temperature to rise. During this period the cervix is in an upward position and opens up to enable the sperm to pass through and meet the egg. It also gets soft with the secretion of the cervical fluid. The duration of the follicular phase varies from one person to another, but for a menstrual cycle of 28 days it lasts about 14 days.

At the end of the follicular phase estrogen in the blood rises to a certain level. In the meantime, LH (luteinizing hormone) makes a sudden surge, causing the follicle to burst for ovulation[3] (releasing the egg). The released egg is sent to the uterus via the fallopian tubes.

If the egg in the tubes meets a sperm ejaculated during sexual intercourse, fertilization will take place. The fertilized embryo then sets off on a journey of 7 days to the uterus by going through a simultaneous self-division, until it nests in the uterus. And this is how a pregnancy starts.

Luteal Phase

If conception does not occur, the luteal phase starts after ovulation, and this phase lasts until the menstrual bleeding. In addition to estrogen, progesterone hormone is secreted during this period by "corpus luteum" (yellow body), the substance left behind by the ruptured follicle. The main role of this hormone is to enable the fertilized egg to cling into uterus, if the released egg gets fertilized.

While the follicular phase varies from one woman to another, depending on the duration of her menstrual cycle, the luteal phase is usually a fixed term of 14 days. Understanding the phases of the menstrual cycle is important to identify the period when you are able to conceive. In light of this information, there are a few ways to figure out the time frame in which you are most prone to conception.

Calendar: If you have regular menstrual periods, the simplest method is to count the days to identify the timing of ovulation. When you count from the first day of your last

---

[3]Ovulation day is roughly 14 days before the start of the menstrual bleeding in a woman who has regular periods. This is the most practical method of determining the ovulation day.

menstrual period, you can determine your most fertile period for conceiving a baby.

Body Temperature: A rise in body temperature is an indication of your most fertile window, because progesterone elevates body temperature. If you take your temperature the first thing in the morning after waking up, and if possible at the same time every day, you may identify the shift in temperature and pinpoint the timing of your ovulation.

Your body temperature is lower (36-36.3°C or 96.8-97.3°F) during the first two weeks of your menstrual cycle, due to the presence of estrogen. Increasing progesterone raises the body temperature so as to provide a warm environment for the fertilized egg instantaneous with ovulation. The temperature increases by at least 0.4-0.6 °C and stays that way after ovulation for the rest of the cycle, or until the beginning of the next cycle. When you observe a temperature increase, you may assume that you have ovulated.

Cervical Fluid: Body temperature indicates ovulation time only. When the temperature goes up, it means the ovulation process has started. But you should not lose sight of other signals, such as cervical fluid. According to many experts, monitoring cervical fluid is a very accurate means of determining the time when you are most likely to get pregnant. There may be continuous discharge, but the ideal period for the sperm to reach the egg is when the discharge is clear, elastic and slippery.

DAY	BODY TEMPERATURE	OBSERVATIONS
1		
2		
3		
4		
5		
6		
7		
8		
9		
10		
11		
12		
13		
14		
15		
16		
17		
18		
19		
20		
21		
22		
23		
24		
25		
26		
27		
28		
29		

Normally, if a woman's cervical fluid, which comes from the uterus, is similar to egg white in consistency, this is a sign of the ovulation cycle or an imminent ovulation. This type of fluid increases in volume during ovulation. Cervical fluid that is slippery, elastic and thin is of an ideal consistency to enable sperm to pass through the cervix. According to research, the structure of this mucus is an excellent indicator of fertility.

Position of the Cervix: Early in the menstrual cycle, the cervix is low and hard. As we explained earlier, it rises, gets softer and opens slightly over time. While we can check the cervix by hand, symptoms such as discomfort in the lower body and occasional one-sided sharp aches can help to identify this phase.

- Is my period today?
- Do I feel sensitive / achy in the abdomen?
- How do I feel? Tired, energetic?
- Do I feel premenstrual tension or stress?
- How is my cervical position?
- Do I have any discharge? If yes, what color and what is its consistency?

You can fill in the sample table in the book to gain a clear understanding of your most fertile period. By doing so over a few months, you will easily discover the specifics of your own cycle. Please fill in the table starting with the first day of your menstrual period. Watch out for other signs by asking the following questions and note your observations on the table after recording your body temperature, right after waking up.

To record your answers to these questions, add notes in the right column of the table such as: “sticky white discharge in the morning,” “sharp pain in the right side of my abdomen in the afternoon,” or “second day of my period, fatigue,” etc

.

GETTING READY FOR PREGNANCY

Now that you have learned about the factors affecting the conception process and fertility signals, let's take a glance at what you need to do when you start planning for pregnancy.

1. Checkup: Consult your doctor and get checked for physical conditions such as cysts, your cervical health, and any infections that can lead to infertility, as mentioned earlier. Have your hormone levels measured and get treated if need be. If there are any medications you are taking on a regular basis, you may want to discuss this with your doctor. You should not ignore the importance of oral health and get any treatments you need now; some kinds of dental treatment aren't recommended during pregnancy and nursing.

2. Stopping birth control: Stop using contraception such as birth control pills or condoms; have your intrauterine device removed if there is one.

3. Vitamin supplement: Start taking supplements such as folic acid and vitamin B.

4. Exercise: If you are not already exercising, it could be beneficial to start a light exercise plan. You can enhance your physical health by doing simple exercises such as taking a walk, swimming and yoga.

5. Positive thinking: You need to let go of negative thoughts in your life to get psychologically ready for motherhood. Try to spare some time for yourself and do things that make you happy. Don't get too hung up on problems. If need be, ask for support from your social circle. Regulating your sleep patterns, taking frequent breaks, and reflecting on your dreams and hopes will be good for you. Another positive thinking exercise would be translating all negative language patterns into positive ones during speaking or writing. For instance, say "let it be easy" instead of "let it be not difficult." Try keeping your speech positive, and you'll see what great change it can make in your life.

6. Stop harmful habits: Smoking, alcohol, caffeinated drinks, off-the-shelf food products, products with chemical content... First of all, make a list of all the harmful things in your lifestyle. It's very important to purify your body and your home and to get ready for the new life that lies ahead. You are starting a brand-new life and your home will soon have a little member. What kind of parents does that little one deserves? What kind of life you will provide for him? The lifestyle changes you make for your child will enhance the quality of your own life and make you a more strong-minded, resilient, disciplined and steadfast person. Smoking and alcohol affect men adversely to the same extent they affect women. Depending on the frequency of smoking, sperm count and sperm motility decline, and functional abnormality and mutations can occur. For this reason, couples trying to conceive should avoid smoking and drinking, and this is equally valid for both partners, regardless of their gender.

7. Weight: Being considerably underweight or overweight affects your fertility. To reach your ideal weight, you first need to question why you are at that particular weight and find the underlying cause. Any chance you are eating unnecessarily or losing your appetite whenever you feel blue? Do you consume high-fat food and sweets, or do you have the habit of eating late? Do you notice that you put on weight more easily when you eat certain things? Before doing anything else, you should try to get rid of your negative thoughts regarding your weight. Instead of saying "I cannot lose weight" or "I tried everything, and nothing has worked," you need to say, "I am changing my weight set point with minor lifestyle changes." Please do not forget that life is actually a series of moments, and it is possible to achieve great outcomes by making small changes! If you are in the habit of exaggerating issues, focus on plans that only involve the next 2 to 3 hours. For example, take a look at your diet list and just tell yourself, "I will try this until noon, and this is a piece of cake for me." Then divide the day into three or four parts by telling yourself, "I will now tolerate this until 4 in the afternoon," and do not let anything distract you from your focus. Dividing a big goal into smaller parts will help you psychologically, and as you succeed in implementing the diet, your new eating habits will be incorporated into your daily routine and you will begin to follow your new way of eating as if on autopilot. If you do happen to fail in one part of it, keep in mind that it was only one of the time slots and you can be successful in the rest. Forgive yourself and continue on the path with new determination. I assure you that your palate and perspective will change over this period. After you start eating healthy, you will find yourself asking this question about the pizza you once ate heartily: "How come I liked this pizza in the past?" and you will be aware of the heaviness it creates in your stomach.

8. Stop excessive dieting: Being on a very low-calorie diet is also a risk factor for infertility. Some studies indicate that an excessive diet leads to a decline in men's ability to have sex and in their sperm motility. Excessive dieting lowers the chance of pregnancy by reducing estrogen and testosterone levels in women and men respectively.

9. Pay attention to your nutrition: Ensure that your food intake contains sufficient quantities of folic acid, zinc, selenium, vitamin E, vitamin B6 and magnesium. Vitamin B6 maintains hormonal balance by eliminating menstrual irregularity. Your iron level should also be at a healthy limit. Vitamin C and E enhance sperm quality in men and obviate hormonal irregularities in women. Zinc and selenium are important vitamins to increase sperm quantity. Lastly, you will learn how to rearrange your kitchen in upcoming sections of the book.

10. Do not use antibiotics and pain relievers in an uninformed manner: Certain pain relievers inhibit prostaglandin hormone in women if they are used during the ovulation period, and this lowers the chance of pregnancy. Misuse of antibiotics sets the stage for fungal infections by interfering with vaginal flora[4]. This, in turn, affects the ability of sperm to fertilize the egg by reducing its motility.

11. Have regular sexual intercourse: Regular sexual intercourse, considered the most important factor in overcoming infertility, increases the chance that sperm will meet the egg and pregnancy will occur. The more regularly you have intercourse, the higher your chance of pregnancy will be.

12. Try to establish regular sleep patterns: People who have irregular sleep patterns have lower levels of a hormone called melatonin. This hormone has positive effects on antioxidant and reproductive functions. The fertility capacity of women with low melatonin secretion is weaker. It is critical that you maintain good sleep routines while trying to

---

[4] **Vaginal flora*:** Harmless micro-organisms in the vagina.

conceive. Going to bed and waking up at the same time every day, with at least eight hours of sleep, will increase your chance of pregnancy.

13. Do not postpone motherhood for the sake of career: It's important to plan for pregnancy before the age of 35, as advanced age is considered an important risk factor for infertility. Fertility is at its peak between the ages of 18 and 30. A woman's fertility capacity starts to decline after 35. Factors related to education and career, economic reasons, and changes to marriage practices have led to an increase in maternal age over the past three decades. The live birth rate decreases in a meaningful way with advanced maternal age.

14. Keep away from environmentally hazardous materials: Scientific research indicates that many environmentally hazardous chemical materials are linked with infertility, pregnancy loss and birth defects. Pesticides, plastics, cleaning materials, and even makeup materials cause many problems ranging from allergy to hormonal imbalances to fertility issues and cancer. The harmful substances that cause hormonal disorders in women can also increase the risk of infertility.

IDEAL WEIGHT TABLE FOR WOMEN								
Age	15-16	17-19	20-24	25-29	30-39	40-49	50-59	60-69
Height	lbs	lbs	lbs	lbs	lbs	lbs	lbs	lbs
4'-9"	97	99	101	106	115	121	123	126
4'-10"	99	101	103	108	117	123	126	128
4'-11"	101	103	106	112	119	126	128	130
4'-12"	103	106	108	112	115	128	130	130
5'-0"	106	108	110	115	117	119	132	132
5'-1"	110	110	115	117	126	132	134	134
5'-2"	110	112	115	119	126	132	137	137
5'-3"	115	117	119	121	130	137	141	141
5'-4"	117	119	121	126	132	141	143	145
5'-5"	121	123	126	130	134	143	148	150
5'-6"	126	128	130	134	141	150	154	154
5'-7"	128	130	132	137	143	152	157	157
5'-8"	132	134	137	141	145	154	161	161
5'-9"	137	139	141	143	150	159	163	163
5'-10"		145	148	150	157	168	172	
5'-11"		148	150	152	159	170	174	
5'-12"		152	154	159	163	174	179	
6'-0"		154	157	161	165	176	181	
Age	15-16	17-19	20-24	25-29	30-39	40-49	50-59	60-69

IDEAL WEIGHT TABLE FOR WOMEN								
Age	15-16	17-19	20-24	25-29	30-39	40-49	50-59	60-69
Height	lbs	lbs	lbs	lbs	lbs	lbs	lbs	lbs
4'-9"	97	99	101	106	115	121	123	126
4'-10"	99	101	103	108	117	123	126	128
4'-11"	101	103	106	112	119	126	128	130
4'-12"	103	106	108	112	115	128	130	130
5'-0"	106	108	110	115	117	119	132	132
5'-1"	110	110	115	117	126	132	134	134
5'-2"	110	112	115	119	126	132	137	137
5'-3"	115	117	119	121	130	137	141	141
5'-4"	117	119	121	126	132	141	143	145
5'-5"	121	123	126	130	134	143	148	150
5'-6"	126	128	130	134	141	150	154	154
5'-7"	128	130	132	137	143	152	157	157
5'-8"	132	134	137	141	145	154	161	161
5'-9"	137	139	141	143	150	159	163	163
5'-10"		145	148	150	157	168	172	
5'-11"		148	150	152	159	170	174	
5'-12"		152	154	159	163	174	179	
6'-0"		154	157	161	165	176	181	
Age	15-16	17-19	20-24	25-29	30-39	40-49	50-59	60-69

IDEAL WEIGHT CALCULATOR BASED ON AGE AND HEIGHT

According to the ideal weight calculator, a person's state of being underweight, overweight or obese is indicated by the following BMI (body mass index) values:

MAN (BMI)	WOMAN (BMI)	Explanation
Below 20.7	Below 19.1	Underweight
Between 20.7-26.4	Between 19.1-25.8	Ideal weight
26.5-27.8	25.9-27.3	Plump; chubby
27.9-31.1	27.4-32.2	Borderline; overweight
31.2-45.4	32.3-44.8	Overweight and obese
Above 45.4	44.8 and above	Dangerously obese, possible health problems

Formula for Ideal Weight Calculation Based on Height:

Male height:1.82 meters

182-150=32

32/4=8

We add 100 to the result (100+8= 108) and subtract it from height (182-108). This formula indicates "74 kilograms" as the ideal weight of the person. The ideal weight is lower for women than men.

Ideal Weight Calculation Based on Age:

Please check the following BMI values to calculate the ideal weight for your age. Example: A person who is 24 years old with a weight of 71 kilograms and a height of 1.76 meters has a BMI of 23 and he is at an ideal weight. The following is the BMI chart based on age:

Am I at an ideal weight?

Age	Rate of Ideal Weight Based on Age
19-24	19-24 BMI
35-44	21-26 BMI
45-54	22-27 BMI
55-65	23-28 BMI
65	24-29 BMI

To see whether you are at your ideal weight, please see the results below. If you are at a normal weight but seem overweight or underweight, you may have your bone weight and body fat rate measured. Body Mass Index (BMI) results can be explained as follows.

Underweight: People who weigh less than the normal weight for their height and age and whose BMI values are below 20.7 for men and 19.1 for women are described as underweight. Even though being underweight signifies beauty for some, it's important to pay attention to the nutrition plan to avoid being significantly underweight.

Ideal weight: Indicates normal weight based on age and height. Implement a weight maintenance diet to keep your weight within this range.

Chubby, plump: People above a normal weight and whose BMI values are above 26.5 for men and 25.9 for women are often described as chubby or plump.

Overweight: People above their ideal weight. BMIs of 31.2 and 32.3 are borderline for men and women respectively.

Obese: People who are significantly overweight can be described as obese. Obesity can lead to health problems, and urgent weight-loss methods should be adopted with the help of a specialist.

PSYCHOLOGICAL AND MENTAL READINESS FOR THE DIET

The fact that you're expecting to go through a process you have not experienced before does not mean that you are not ready for it. The changes you make in your life for your future baby will gradually prepare you for this process in any case. Let's look at what we can do to transform this process into a more enjoyable and conscious one.

Manage your stress: The Division of Epidemiology, Statistics and Prevention Research (DESPR) of NICHD worked in cooperation with their colleagues at Oxford University in the United Kingdom and measured alpha-amylase levels in the saliva of women who were trying to conceive. This study revealed that women with higher levels of alpha-amylase, which are linked to high stress levels, were less likely to get pregnant than women who had lower concentrations of alpha-amylase. This research suggests that stress lowers the probability of pregnancy.

While stress is the nuisance of our time in many respects, the stress a married couple goes through can even hinder their fertility. Patients undergoing infertility treatment endure severe stress. Such couples are exposed to chronic stress every single month when a treatment fails to yield the desired outcome. Acupuncture, yoga, meditation, massage, deep breathing techniques, praying and visualization can help you overcome this stress. The most obvious feeling that arises from these practices is that of relaxation. Listening to music, taking long walks, exercising, outdoor activity to get some fresh air, or anything that would make you feel good will help you manage your stress.

Read: It is possible to prepare in a better way for this process by reading the relevant magazines, books, and online articles written by specialists. Do not feel anxious about what you learn, just firmly believe that everything will be all right and you will be able to cope with any situation you come across. Keep in mind that you will be holding your baby in your arms at the end of this journey. Each piece of information you gain along the way exists to serve this purpose. After all, nature psychologically prepares people in the best way for this process by changing hormonal balances.

Consult: If something occupies your mind, ask your doctor and friends who have gone through this process. You don't need to rediscover everything for yourself if you can draw on the experiences of women who have traveled the path of motherhood before. For this reason, meet a mother each week to chat, and turn that into a routine. Meeting with mothers can motivate you better during your pregnancy-preparation process than meeting with single friends.

Meditate: Many people perceive meditation as an attempt to stop the mind from thinking and give it up after one or two tries, saying "I cannot quiet my mind, I cannot do this." As a matter of fact, meditation is not quieting the mind. Most of us think we need to strive and focus to be successful. However, the more we strive, the tenser we become, and this seems to be a barrier to success. In fact, meditation is a training exercise that strengthens your mind just the way physical exercise strengthens your body. You will experience the anxious, nervous voice in your mind gradually calming down and becoming more positive and peaceful as you stick to your meditation practice. If you are not close to a meditation center and cannot budget any money for this, just start meditating by using online videos or relevant books. Spare a half-hour for meditation daily and do it regularly for the first 21 days. Even if you do not observe a change initially, you will be surprised to see how you will be in tune with the flow of life as you keep up with your meditation practice.

Develop mindfulness: As of now, you have to think for two rather than one. If you drink a lot of coffee or smoke, remember your future baby when your hand reaches out for such things and act accordingly. The same holds true when you feel sad or stressed! You might also save some baby pictures on your phone and occasionally look at them to get motivated.

Pray: Regardless of how much we would like to manage the process, our sphere of influence is limited in life. Therefore, leave the rest to God, with relief, after you do all you can to prepare. Make it your intention to see, hear and know what is best for you, your baby and family. It will be in your best interest to have a faithful reliance during this process.

Talk to your spouse: Spare some time to talk together about your shared dreams involving your future baby and family. Keep in mind that he also needs to get psychologically ready as part of this process. You can help and direct him.

Prepare your physical condition and plan for your future: To feel financially strong, you need to plan ahead. For instance, how will you deal with your job, which health insurance will you use, and who will help you to take care of the baby after birth? This does not always have to be a baby caretaker. Your mother, mother-in-law, neighbor, or a colleague from work can help with this. Some moms band together in the spirit of the "solidarity of motherhood" and share child care duties when one or the other is busy.

Get support from a personal development coach: Sometimes women cannot get pregnant due to wrong codings in their subconscious, even if they seem to desire a pregnancy. If there is no physical barrier and you still cannot get pregnant, you may benefit from therapy methods such as EFT (Emotional Freedom Technique) and Family Constellation to clean up locks in your subconscious. You can gain a lot from methods such as Sedona (letting go) or Ho'oponopono (law of attraction), which you can implement by yourself.

Ho'oponopono
Ho'oponopono, according to Md. Hew Len, is "a cleaning that aims to correct an error in one's subconscious." Everyone must implement this on their own. The essence of Ho'oponopono is to understand that we are responsible for anything that happens to us in life, no matter what it is. When you have a problem, the only thing you need to do is to say "I am fully responsible for this problem. I love you. Thank you. Please forgive me."

Sedona Method

The Sedona Method is a practice of letting go. Life coach, instructor and consultant Kemal Islamoglu describes the method as follows: "Our brain codes everything through vision, smell, emotion and sound. Regardless of what our negative memories are, when we catch their codes, we can solve the problem by letting them go, just like a balloon lifting from within us. When the balloon flies, some residue will be left for sure. We need to gather this residue, turn it into a balloon and make it fly as well. We should do this again and again. This practice will thoroughly clean the residue after a certain period and the disturbance will go away to a major extent. This is how the method is applied: first close your eyes and focus on the particular toxic emotion you are currently feeling. Then, you find where that emotion is and start describing it based on some questions such as: What color is it? What shape? How heavy or big is it?

After you clearly picture the feeling in your mind, you need to focus on letting it go. Are you ready to let it go? When can you let it go? Then you focus on getting that emotion out of your body. Some mentally leave their toxic emotions on the floor by releasing them from the tips of their toes. Some throw them far away; some dispel them by crushing them thoroughly. After that, you redirect your attention to yourself and make sure nothing of the negative emotion is left behind in your body; that you are totally purified of it.

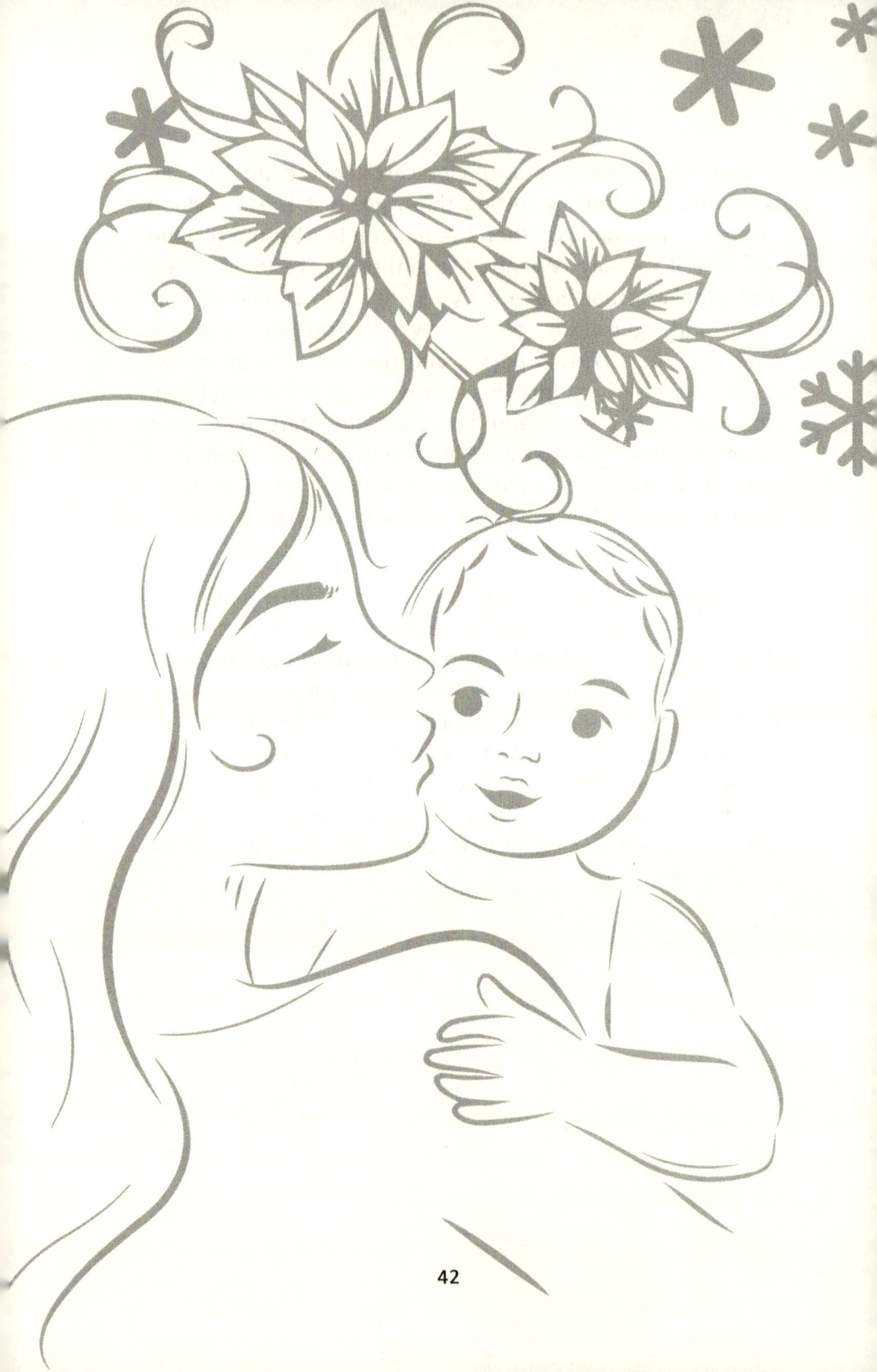

Chapter Three

PRE-CONCEPTION NUTRITION

Anyone can practice the proper way of eating to encourage natural conception, regardless of their specific fertility problem, age, income or time limitations. We all eat. So, why not eat in a way that will support fertility?

Did you know that what you eat today will affect the health quality of your egg or sperm 90 days later?

A prospective mother's nutritional needs change beginning with the moment of conception. However, detoxifying the body for a certain period and eating carefully before pregnancy are necessary both to increase the chance of pregnancy and to give birth to a healthy baby. **I personally think that the significance of nutrition for fertility is not emphasized enough.** For instance, in England, 500 million euros are spent annually on medical procedures and medications to overcome infertility, but prospective parents are not told that their chances of conception could be increased by proper nutrition. Research conducted in 1995 by Surrey University for the Association for Promotion of Preconceptual Care (Foresight) is striking. The study involved 367 couples who were at an advanced age, diagnosed with infertility, and had experienced a miscarriage requiring a D&C. These couples were put on a special healthy life and diet program, during which they were purified of toxins. Within two years, 81% of these couples who had been diagnosed with infertility were able to have a baby.

Unfortunately, the same attitude is also observed in our country. Fertility-oriented nutrition is a valid approach not only for prospective mothers but also prospective fathers. Studies indicate that even the slightest change, such as both partners taking multivitamin pills, affects sperm quality and healthy ovulation. However, some initial tests are necessary before starting to use multivitamins, to prevent vitamin overload.

Almost all cells in our body go through a life cycle of their own. Cells grow old, die, and are cleared from the system as newly formed cells replace them and take over their tasks. There is a continuous maintenance and repair process in the nerve and muscle cells that cannot be renewed through cellular division, and these cells retain their vitality by being renewed internally. We need new building stones to enable the formation of new cells and to sustain the vitality of the existing ones; and here's where nutrition comes in, providing our body with these building blocks.

Proper nutrition depends on many factors, ranging from selection of ingredients in the preparation stage, to the interaction of food with the enzymes in saliva after we take a bite of something, the digestive functions of the stomach, and interaction of various food items when consumed together. Factors such as the cooking method and the amount consumed also make a difference in the way the body uses the food. So, given these circumstances, what kind of a process should we follow? Let's get started.

What to Consider While Choosing Nutrients

We used to eat all-organic up to about four or five decades ago. But today, many products that are genetically modified, full of chemicals, frozen, or containing harmful chemicals that we are hardly aware of end up on our dining tables. Expelling toxins from our kitchen by weeding out the harmful products and following a healthy diet are two musts, both for our own bodies and for the healthy development of our future babies.

Even though industrialized food production provides more product variety and a greater volume of products, certain chemicals, pesticides, and artificial fertilizers cause the food to grow differently.

In our country, agriculture deemed to be organic is a process in which all stages of production are inspected, and pesticides, artificial fertilizers, hormones and antibiotics are not used in any of these stages; in fact, they are not even available in the production environment. Organic products are more expensive than industrial products, because higher productivity is achieved on farms where chemicals are used on products to rid them of pests. Organically grown fruits and vegetables typically see lower yields, as other living beings in nature also want to feed on organic agricultural products. Accordingly, production costs go up.

The good news is that the number of institutions engaging in organic agriculture is steadily increasing. Still, these products may not always be available everywhere. If you cannot find organic products, your alternative should be GAP (good agricultural practices) certified products.

The institutions established to protect consumer rights in this regard are approved by the Ministry of Agriculture and Rural Affairs, and they receive special control authorization. In Turkey, there are about 25 institutions that have this authorization document. These institutions inspect producers and issue a permit that allows them to label their products as organic. You can go online to reach the inspecting institutions and the producers who have filed an application to these institutions.

What to Consider While Making Food Choices

Please consume products that are in season. Fruits and vegetables grown seasonally taste and smell much better and have better nutritional value than those grown in greenhouses. By choosing such products, you will be able to eat a food item when it has the highest nutritional value.

Try to consume wild-caught fish instead of farmed fish. Wild-caught fish have higher quality of meat and nutritional values, as they get their nutrients from a much larger area in the sea. Cold-water fish are preferable thanks to their nutritional value and the cleanliness of water from which they're harvested, even if these fish are imported from overseas.

Choose organic meat from grass-fed cattle. The meat of traditionally raised cattle contains high levels of hormones and antibiotics, which will curb estrogen. On the other hand, the meat of grass-fed animals is a wonderful source of essential fatty acids, because its saturated fat content is low, and it is a great source of protein. A research shows some connection between high red meat consumption and endometriosis. For this reason, if you are suffering from endometriosis, you need to reduce the amount of red meat you eat.

Try to buy free-range organic chicken. Traditionally raised chicken is kept in dirty, overly crowded coops and fed with genetically modified, nonorganic stuff. Always look for "cage free," "free-range" or "organic" descriptions on the labels. It is also best to buy the chicken from a local farm.

Getting Ready for the Motherhood Diet

Now let us talk about the Motherhood Diet. The basis of this diet is the balanced consumption of all food groups, namely carbohydrates, proteins and fats. We have tried to choose food items that are slowly digested. These foods will keep blood sugar balanced after and between meals. Slowly digested food prevents insulin and glucagon hormones from rapidly turning our food intake into sugar. Insulin resistance declines once blood sugar gets balanced, which in turn reduces the probability of hormonal and ovarian problems. What is essential is not to consume *zero* sugar or carbohydrates, but rather to keep blood sugar from fluctuating considerably during the day, and eventually to maintain a good hormonal balance.

Before talking about how you should consume each of the food groups, let's name the items you should take out of your kitchen.

Foods to Avoid Strictly	Replacement Alternatives
Instant soup	Homemade soups prepared by using fresh ingredients
Pizza	
Processed meat products such as pepperoni, salami and hot dogs	
Off-the-shelf jam and marmalade	Homemade sugar-free jam or
Off-the-shelf fruit juice	Fresh fruit juice, compote, fruit
Off-the-shelf sauces	
Off-the-shelf desserts	
Off-the-shelf breakfasts	Food that is suitable for your
Snacks such as chocolate, chips,	Nuts, fresh or dried fruits
White bread, pasta, rice	Whole-wheat bread, bulgur
Early fruits and vegetables	Seasonal fruits and vegetables
Industrial eggs	Village eggs
Industrial yoghurt	Homemade yoghurt prepared
Margarine and similar oleos	Extra-virgin olive oil, fresh butter
Canned food with additives	Homemade preserves
Farm fish, mussels that absorb	Fresh salt-water fish

It is important to banish the food items in the left column from your kitchen before you start your diet. That's because the only way to keep yourself away from all the factors that will distract you or make you go back to your old habits is to get them out of the house. Instead, fill your cupboards and fridge with healthy products. Those who have a food intolerance should use substitute products for any items in the right column.

FOOD GROUPS

We need three main building blocks to meet the energy requirements of our body: proteins, carbohydrates and fats. Each of the building blocks carries out different tasks. Let's have a closer look at these three building blocks and food groups.

Carbohydrates

In the previous chapter we mentioned that an insulin upsurge raises testosterone by affecting globulin, which is the hormone carrier in the blood, and this affects fertility adversely. Carbohydrates also have a bad reputation in the same way, because they rapidly increase blood sugar after digestion. So, does this mean we should not consume any carbohydrates?

Professor Md. Canan Karatay has waged a war on sugar in her books and on the TV programs where she was featured. She describes sugar as the most dangerous substance of the century and even talks about it as a form of poison. While many scientists support that position, some come up with opposite conclusions. So, which perspective is true?

Our body is a structure undergoing a continuous process of demolition and rebuilding, with a fabulous balance. While millions of cells die and are removed by cleaner cells, millions of cells are produced simultaneously to replace these cells. Cancer cells, on the other hand, are cells that continuously self-divide, migrate to other parts of the body where they should not be, secrete stimulant chemicals, and have the ability to affect their region and the related system negatively.

Well, would you be surprised if I told you that cancer cells develop even in a healthy person from time to time, but the body recognizes and clears them during the development stage? Sometimes intracellular mechanisms, and at other times extracellular events, prevent these cells from developing and growing; in a nutshell, the body protects itself.

The keyword in the above paragraph is "healthy." Even a healthy individual may have cancer cells. But how can we describe a person who has cancer cells in their body as healthy? Here's where a very important concept comes in, that of "balance." As long as the systems in our body are in balance, we can call ourselves healthy. So, we can describe a person as healthy if cancer cells occasionally develop but get cleared without causing any health problems. This is a process that happens in every single person.

The same holds true for nutrition. Carbohydrates, or sugar, are the single energy source of certain cell types in our body, and for this reason it is not very accurate to describe sugar as "poison." Once again, balance is an important element. Sugar is the easiest and most efficient source for meeting the body's energy demands. In other words, giving up sugar totally is not actually possible. As a matter of fact, certain cells, such as the brain cells, love sugar so much that they have been structured to get their energy supply only from sugar.

No food item in nature is purely carbohydrate, fat, or protein. In all living beings, almost all forms of nourishment involve these three building blocks. A food item cannot be made up of solely carbohydrates, or proteins, or fats. Every single food item consists of these three basic components or their subcomponents in some way, because all three of them are together necessary for a living being to sustain life. For example, a steak has three of these components, but its highest content is protein. An apple, on the other hand, has more carbohydrate.

What variations do we see if we look at carbohydrate, fat or protein components more closely? In other words, does every single carbohydrate, fat or protein component have the same content as their counterparts in a different food? Let's put it this way: Is the carbohydrate we get from apple the same as the carbohydrate we get from lettuce, or is the protein we get from turkey the same as the protein we get from an egg? Or do they differ from each other?

There are different classes of carbohydrates, and as you might have guessed, carbohydrates are a little different in each food item. As the main effect of carbohydrates is to elevate blood sugar, we classify them according to their effects on blood sugar and metabolism, rather than their biochemical structures.

Glycemic load is a determinative factor in terms of carbohydrate consumption. It refers to the average value of how quickly your blood sugar rises, given the particular food and how much of it you consume in a meal. One should avoid foods with a high glycemic load and prefer those with a low glycemic load. When we consume food with a lower glycemic load, our blood sugar rises in a more stable way, spikes do not occur in our insulin level, and as a result our reproductive hormones are not affected negatively.

In conclusion, it is necessary to consume food that does not cause a rapid rise in blood sugar, or that has a low glycemic index, while implementing the Motherhood Diet. We will meet the carbohydrate needs of our body with low glycemic index foods such as fruits and vegetables, whole grains and legumes, instead of bread, pasta, rice, pastries and potatoes, which have a high glycemic index. Low glycemic foods are also beneficial for patients suffering from polycystic ovary syndrome, as they do not cause a sudden increase in blood sugar and keep it balanced.

Below is a table showing glycemic index values for various foods:

High Glycemic Index (100-70)	Moderate Glycemic Index (69-50)	Low Glycemic Index (49-0)
All refined and processed foods	Dark bread, whole wheat bread	Whole rye bread
Sugar, saccharose, maltose, glucose, glucose syrup	Oatmeal	Legumes (chickpeas, beans, lentil)
Anything with added sugar	Brown rice	Carrots
Starch	Beets	Cabbage
Corn, corn flakes, popcorn, corn flour, muesli (breakfast cereals)	Melon	Artichoke, celery
Fruit juices	Raisins, dates, dried figs	Eggplant
White bread, sandwich, toast, hamburger, pitta, bagel	Apricot	Zucchini
Anything with white flour (white rice, white pasta)	Chestnut	Scallions and onions
Honey	Semolina	Broccoli
Potatoes	Foods on the border of 50 GI	Pepper (all colors)
Cooked carrot	Whole wheat bread and flour	Cucumber
Millet, millet drink (boza)	Bulgur	Any kind of greens that can be eaten raw (lettuce, mint, parsley, dill, basil, oregano, sweet basil)
Pumpkin	Peas	Mushroom
Watermelon, mulberry, fresh figs, banana	Grapes, kiwi	

Based on the feedback I get from my patients, I know that the biggest challenge you will face after you start this diet will be eliminating rice pilaf, pasta and pastries, which have a high glycemic index and create a feeling of fullness. Leaving the dining table chock-full is a social habit of ours. You might think that leaving the table partially hungry will not make you happy, or you might even say, "I cannot feel full unless I eat bread." Such comments just reveal a psychological fixation. Thoughts like *no meal is complete without bread* or *pilaf is the must-have side dish to haricot beans or chickpeas* lead to the addition of another dish that will fill your stomach. White bread does cause a feeling of fullness due to the volume it occupies, but this lasts only temporarily. Your body will digest the bread within a short period of time, elevating blood sugar rapidly and causing insulin to be secreted right afterward, leading to a rapid drop in your blood sugar. As a result, you will get hungry again within two hours. And when you become hungry again, you will also crave something rich in carbohydrates and keep this vicious cycle going. Whole grains are recommended on the diet lists for many diseases, including diabetes, just as they are on the fertility diet, because of their health benefits. Whole-grain bread is recommended not only to meet carbohydrate needs and create a feeling of

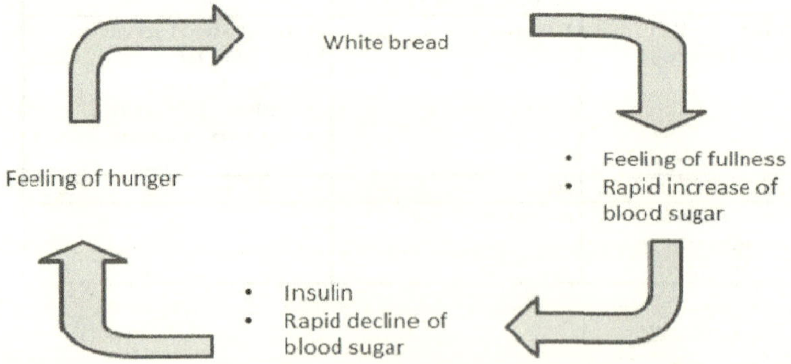

fullness, but also for its richness of vitamins and minerals, and primarily for its fiber content.

To feel pleasantly satisfied, we need to consume high-protein foods that will pass through the stomach slowly; in other words, we should consume food that is digested more slowly. By doing so, blood sugar will increase more gradually and steadily, and we will feel full for a longer period of time. In a nutshell, choose small amounts of whole grains or oat bread rather than white bread; replace white rice with brown rice; and eat bulgur instead of pasta.

Fats

Fat is a sine qua non for our body. If our body cannot produce certain fatty acids, we will have to get these from somewhere, as they're needed for certain vital functions. For years, a lot has been said negatively about fats: that they were very harmful, they should not be consumed, would cause atherosclerosis and weight gain, make your body unhealthy, and so on. In fact, cholesterols and fatty acid compounds in the content of fats are among the important structures needed by the human body for certain vital functions. Refraining from all fats is neither practically possible nor healthy. In other words, while fats in and of themselves are not harmful for our body, a deficiency of fats can damage our bodies. Therefore, there is no point in hating fats. The reason doctors all over the world recommend reducing fat consumption is that fats are often improperly used in the diet.

As Professor Md. Canan Karatay also advocates, fats are essential and protective nutrients. It is necessary to get fatty acids such as Omega3 and 6 from external sources, as our bodies can't produce them. Omega3 (EPA and DHA) is produced by alfa-linolenic acid in our body. We know that Omega3 and 6, which may be obtained in good quantities from walnuts, hazelnuts, spinach, fish oil, broccoli, sunflower seeds, corn, soy and grains, carry out critical tasks such as supporting the immune system and protecting the body against cancer. Fats also take on tasks like vitamin D absorption and protection of sex hormones. So, which fats should we take out of our lives, and which ones should we consume in a conscious and balanced manner?

Fats are divided into three groups: trans fats, saturated, and unsaturated fats.

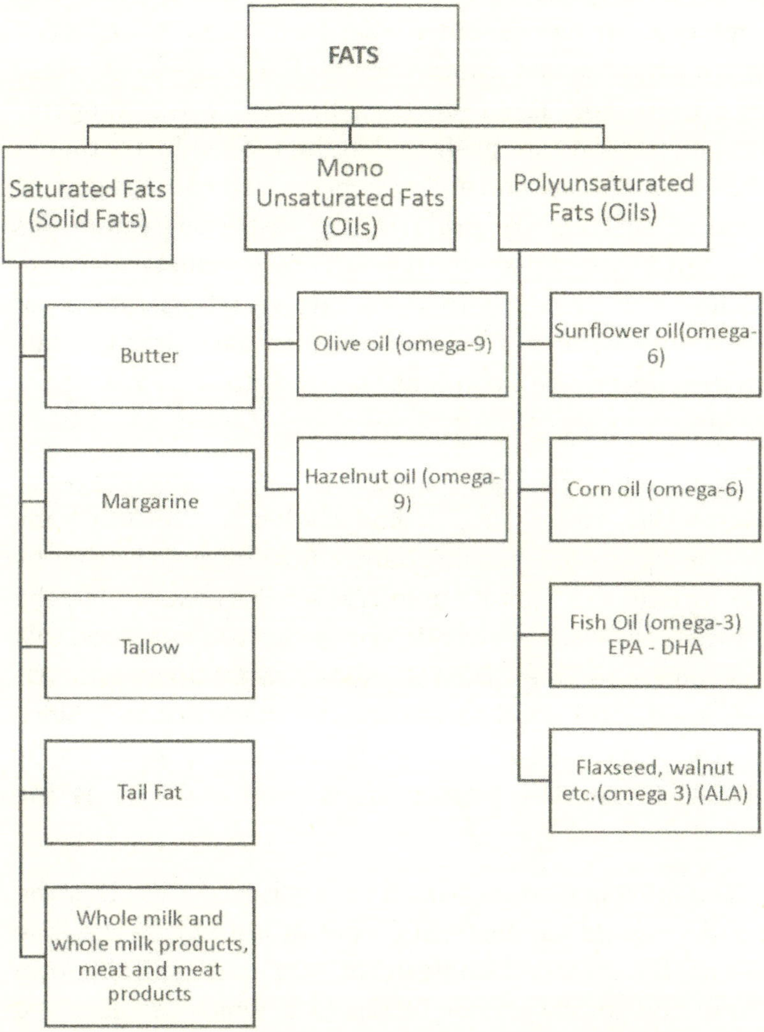
FATS
Saturated Fats (Solid Fats)
Mono Unsaturated Fats (Oils)
Polyunsaturated Fats (Oils)
Butter
Margarine
Tallow
Tail Fat
Whole milk and whole milk products, meat and meat products
Olive oil (omega-9)
Hazelnut oil (omega-9)
Sunflower oil(omega-6)
Corn oil (omega-6)
Fish Oil (omega-3) EPA - DHA
Flaxseed, walnut etc.(omega 3) (ALA)

Trans Fats

Trans fats are the most dangerous group among fats and responsible for the "bad and dangerous" reputation that fats have garnered over the years. These are fats that do not exist in nature but derive from chemically forced compounds of unsaturated fats and hydrogen. In other words, these are "fats that are saturated with hydrogen." Hydrogenated fats are preferred in the food industry thanks to their affordability and ability to be reused without getting spoiled. Trans fats are preferred by fast-food restaurants and often in off-the-shelf convenience products, because food items produced with trans fats won't go rancid for many months. There is a high chance the chocolate you buy from the supermarket contains trans fats to sustain a longer shelf life.

This type of fat, which is very advantageous commercially, raises LDL, or bad cholesterol, in the body after it is digested. Trans fats harm the body even further by lowering HDL, the "good" cholesterol that is absorbed by the cell structure. A patient of mine once showed me blood test results and asked me: "Doctor, my HDL went up and my LDL went down; do I need to change the medications?" Since that day, I have been explaining this to my patients by labelling HDL as the blessed cholesterol and LDL as the damned cholesterol.

The most important aspect of fats is to ensure that the blessed, or good, cholesterol is kept at normal levels while lowering the damned cholesterol. We must refrain from harmful and totally artificial trans fats, which increase the damned cholesterol while lowering the blessed cholesterol.

Fats are very sensitive. When they are exposed to excessive heat, their structures change and turn into trans fats. You can use unsaturated fats, in other words vegetable oils, such as olive oil, by paying attention to the oil's source and quality; but you should be especially careful not to burn the oil. You should not use frying oil any more than once. Of course, it is best for your health to boil or steam some food items rather than frying them.

Trans fats also create a hormonal imbalance by increasing insulin resistance. Please read the labels carefully on off-the-shelf convenience products and exclude those containing trans fats, as well as fast-food products, from your diet.

Saturated Fats

Animal fats, whose occasional consumption is harmless, are the solid fat derivatives that remain firm at room temperature and are present in foods such as meat, butter, milk and cheese. In saturated fats, the carbon atoms in the fat are encircled by the maximum number of hydrogen atoms they can hold; to put it differently, they are saturated with hydrogen atoms.

It is not possible to get saturated fats out of our lives, nor is it necessary. The focus should be on not consuming them excessively, or alone. As long as they are consumed together with unsaturated, or healthy, fats, saturated fats can be used in our food. Eating these fats excessively will elevate LDL and cause vascular occlusion. This, in turn, will affect fertility negatively.

Unsaturated Fats

The most essential oils for health and fertility are within this category. Unsaturated fats are in liquid form at room temperature and can be further classified as either "monounsaturated" or "polyunsaturated." While monounsaturated fats can be produced by our body in other fatty acids, polyunsaturated fats cannot; for this reason, we need to get them from outside sources. Monounsaturated fats are in liquid form at room temperature. Olive oil is one example. Other vegetable oils such as hazelnut oil and almond oil are also in this category. Monounsaturated fats are healthy. They lower LDL, which can cause obstruction in arteries, and increase HDL, which is necessary for nerve cells and preventive against cardiovascular diseases. Therefore, cardiovascular disease specialists and cardiologists recommend olive oil to their patients.

Monounsaturated fats prevent an increase of insulin resistance by raising insulin sensitivity. In the previous chapter, I underlined the fact that the probability of conception drops when insulin resistance increases. For this reason, consumption of monounsaturated fats such as olive and other vegetable oils is beneficial for our reproductive health. The most harmless ones are olive oil, canola oil, other liquid oils and vegetable oils.

As you know, olives are abundantly produced, especially along the Aegean coast. The highest quality olive oil brands in the world come from the Mediterranean region as well. Most countries are not as lucky as we are in this aspect. Countries on the Mediterranean coast tend to use a lot of olive oil in their cooking, due to their climate and food cultures. This is one of the most important reasons for the long and healthy lifespans of Mediterranean people!

We know that olive oil comes in various kinds. In some types, trans fats can form due to the application of heat to obtain the product, and these trans fats can be harmful to our health. Healthy olive oil is obtained through the traditional method of cold-pressing.

I mentioned earlier that polyunsaturated fats cannot be produced by our bodies and must be obtained from food. The most important -among the polyunsaturated fats are Omega3 and Omega6. These are available in considerable amounts in cold-water fish such as salmon, sardines and tuna. They can also be obtained from some vegetable sources such as sunflower, corn and soy oils. Consuming polyunsaturated fats is also important in terms of fertility. These fats yield positive effects just like monounsaturated fats, by reducing the LDL that causes obstructions in the circulatory system. As our body does not produce polyunsaturated fats, we must obtain them from the right sources and in sufficient amounts.

Being careful with your fish consumption is important, because some fish may contain mercury. In summary, the structure of fats should be unimpaired, healthy and pure—in other words, natural—and fats should be used properly in cooking. You should use oils at an appropriate temperature and not allow trans-fat formation by overheating or reheating them.

1	Fats are not a food source you should avoid.
2	We need to consume fats in their natural forms as far as possible.
3	Fats are sensitive substances that are responsive to heat.
4	We must get Omega3 and Omega6 fatty acids from food sources, because our body cannot produce them. It is beneficial to consume food that is rich in both, in order to
5	While olive oil is precious due to its content, we need to take care in using the kind that has not been exposed to
6	Trans fats impact fertility negatively.
7	You can have food items that contain fat as part of your meal. However, calories coming from fat should not
8	Very thin women can have difficulty in getting pregnant and keeping the pregnancy. For this reason, the female

Proteins

Proteins are the main regulatory molecules in our body. These molecules play a key role in many tasks, such as transmission and packaging of molecular information, recognition of external materials, and intercellular communication. A big portion of our DNA, which is what makes us who we are, is where proteins are coded.

Proteins are also composed of building blocks, just like carbohydrates and fats. When we eat a food item that contains protein, our body digests it and breaks down the protein into smaller building blocks called amino acids. Later on, these building blocks are carried to the parts of our body where they are needed. In other words, what we eat becomes a part of us.

The human body creates certain amino acids from scratch, but only a small percentage of the amino acids we need. At the end of the day, people consume vegetables and animal protein to get the necessary amino acids. Therefore, proteins play a key role in our nutrition. Many bodily systems, such as the immune and growth systems, are negatively affected by a protein deficiency. Proteins are also essential for conception. Healthy functioning of the reproductive system may be at stake when there is a protein deficiency. For this reason, consuming a sufficient amount of protein is important for women who are trying to conceive.

Proteins have a more complex structure than fats and carbohydrates, because protein molecules contain a significantly higher number of building blocks. Hundreds of amino acids that are known today can combine in different ways to form proteins. Yet, all proteins do not contain all the known amino acids. In other words, the amino acid content we get from fish is different from the one we get from lamb.

Even though proteins are present at high rates in foods of animal origin such as meat, milk, and cheese, they are also available in vegetables in rich amounts. Amino acids from vegetarian sources and amino acids of animal sources differ from each other. Living beings who feed on plants need to eat a variety of them to get the necessary amino acids.

So, how important is the source of protein? Are animal proteins more valuable than vegetable proteins? Which one should we choose to increase our chances of conception? Animal proteins provide us with a more integral package, as they involve all amino acids. If you eat animal-source proteins, you can get all the amino acids you need in one meal. On the other hand, proteins from vegetarian sources include many amino acids as well, and these foods also serve as a source of vitamins, minerals and fatty acids, which are essential for your body. As a result, if vegetable dishes that are rich in protein are on your weekly menu, you do not have to worry about your protein and amino acid intake, because you have already made a healthy choice.

Perpetual consumption of red meat increases the animal or saturated fat intake that comes with meat, and for this reason it will cause an undesirable increase in LDL. Protein amino acids are also necessary for hormonal balance, to the extent they are necessary for the development of a healthy egg and sperm. Of course, what matters is the amount and type of protein we get. According to the World Health Organization, you can calculate the amount of protein you need by multiplying your weight by 0.8. For example, a woman who weighs 60 kilograms will need 48 grams of protein per day, which is 60x0.8. This figure can vary based on certain conditions, such as being pregnant, nursing a baby, or working at a physically demanding job.

You need to diversify your protein intake as much as possible, just as you should do with other nutrients. Consuming both animal and vegetarian protein sources will enable the transformation of all amino acids that are needed by our body into the right building blocks.

We can draw an analogy between protein and an engineer. An engineer is usually responsible for planning and management in a factory, but at least nominally is able to carry out the tasks of an ordinary production worker. Imagine you're the boss at the factory, and that there is an open spot at the production level of the plant, and you direct the engineer to that spot to do the task of a worker. As the engineer doesn't have sufficient experience for this task, he does the work more slowly and expensively. He also gets tired more quickly as he is used to doing less physical work than the factory worker. He also complains about working conditions and brings up his legal rights in a bid to go back to his own work of planning and management. As the boss of the plant, you end up unable to get the desired productivity out of your engineer, and your factory performance overall declines because there's a gap at the management level.

Protein is like that engineer; it's used mostly in building body structure. When necessary, proteins can also be used as a source of energy, but this isn't the most appropriate use for the body. Our body doesn't use proteins, like the engineer in our story, as a source of energy unless it has to. That's because getting energy from proteins is costly, difficult and inefficient. For this reason, the body uses carbohydrates, better known as "sugar," to meet its energy needs.

Even though sugar and fat, other building blocks that provide our body with energy, are similar to each other, there is a distinction between them. While the body uses sugar for its sudden energy needs, fat is the stored energy source. The body stores excessive sugar as fat to be used for later. The body performs certain processes while transforming sugar into a storable form. This necessitates some extra steps to prepare the fat for energy use in the future. As a result, using fat as a source of energy is not as easy as using sugar. So, the body uses sugar as the primary source of energy.

As I mentioned earlier, our body needs insulin to feed sugar into the cell. This means that the more sweets we consume, the more insulin we produce. Secretion of the insulin hormone at a higher level triggers the stimulation of certain organs and structures, production of other hormones and similar substances, and changes in the body.

Vitamins and Minerals

Do you know that the total mineral content of an adult's body is six percent? A great portion of those minerals, primarily calcium and phosphorus, are the building blocks of the skeleton. While sodium and potassium balance body fluids, iron enables oxygen to be conveyed to the tissues, a process that's necessary to transform nutritional elements into energy. Minerals are also present in the compounds of enzymes that regulate the body and are also used in the body's defense system.

Vitamins, on the other hand, have tremendous effects on us, even though they exist in very small amounts in the body. Studies conducted in the USA show that when couples get multivitamin support, their immune systems become stronger, fertility increases, the possibility of ovulation-related infertility declines, and even the overall infertility risk goes down by 41%. According to a different study, the chance of conception increases with additional diet supplements involving vitex fruit (chaste tree or vitex agnus-castus), green tea, and vitamins E and B6. Studies also indicate that 26% of women who start taking a multivitamin support get pregnant within the first three months, compared to 10% of women who are not on multivitamins.

In addition to vitamin support, we need to pay attention to the vitamin and mineral balance of our food intake. Antioxidants, vitamins and minerals help to protect egg and sperm health. But, before you start taking vitamins like crazy based on this piece of information, I want to add a note of caution. It's important that your vitamin intake be monitored by a doctor. Your blood values should be checked, and it is critical that you only take the vitamins and minerals that are actually needed by your body.

Vitamin B6: Plays a role in regulating blood sugar and hormonal balance. At the same time, it is effective during the luteal phase, which is one of the phases of ovulation in women. Vitamin B6 food sources are fish, liver and green-leafy vegetables.

Vitamin B12: This is a vitamin stored in our liver. It is very important in terms of the structure of erythrocytes, the cells carrying oxygen in the blood. It plays a role in fertilization and the things that happen in the uterus after fertilization and reduces the possibility of a miscarriage. Foods rich in Vitamin B12 are fish and meat. We commonly observe B12 vitamin deficiency in our society. You should consult your doctor to see if there is a deficiency.

Folic Acid: This is the vitamin whose relationship with pregnancy is commonly known. There may be certain birth defects in the baby if the mother has a folic acid deficiency during her pregnancy. These are abnormalities such as heart diseases, cleft lip and palate, and neural tube defects. Mothers with folic acid deficiency have a higher risk of miscarriage and preterm labor. Checking folic acid levels is crucial during pregnancy. Some food sources rich in folic acid are liver, legumes, spinach and bulgur.

Vitamin C: Vitamin C plays a role in the repair of DNA damage. It is very important for the prevention of miscarriages that happen due to chromosomal damage. It is also effective against the ovulation problems that arise in the luteal phase. Vitamin C is found abundantly in citrus fruits, raspberries, tomatoes and peppers.

Vitamin D: This vitamin has one very different feature from the others. Vitamin D needs to be activated by sunlight in order to be used by the body. In other words, if a person does not get enough sunlight, this vitamin, which plays an important role in the functions of reproductive hormones, is not produced sufficiently regardless of the richness of Vitamin D in a person's diet. For this reason, getting out of the house every day, taking a walk, and having skin contact with sunlight are critically important. Ultraviolet sunlight activates Vitamin D. Let me make note of a detail here; ultraviolet light is refracted when it passes through glass and cannot create the effect necessary for activation. So, sunbathing in front of a closed window will not work. You need to go out every day and expose your skin to sun for twenty to thirty minutes, to the best of your ability. Vitamin

D is available in egg, fish and especially cold-water fish. You need to make sure these food items are included in your diet.

Vitamin E: Vitamin E is among the most important antioxidants. It is mostly available in green-leafy vegetables, olives, spinach, and pumpkin and sunflower seeds. Antioxidants prevent deterioration of certain molecular and structural elements that play important roles in our body. Consider antioxidants as a kind of preventive insurance. Following a diet that is rich in antioxidants is highly beneficial for our body.

Coenzyme Q10: It prevents DNA damage that comes from the free oxygen radicals. It is also a molecule that is necessary to generate energy in every single cell. In scientific studies, this enzyme has been observed to enhance egg and sperm health. Coenzyme Q10 is available in fish and red meat. However, diet per se is not sufficient to provide this molecule in the required amount. For this reason, getting supplements is the best option, but you need to consult your doctor first.

Iron: The ovulation cycle is also interrupted in women with iron deficiency. Iron gets integrated into the structure of erythrocytes, which carry oxygen in the blood, and it is an indispensable element in terms of the oxygenation of tissues. Iron deficiency is observed in women in high rates, and it is the major reason of anemia in our country. The ovulation rate in women with iron deficiency increases, while the egg quality decreases. If a woman has trouble conceiving, one of the first questions that need to be answered is whether there is enough iron in her body.

Liver, red meat, fish, soybeans and grapes are foods rich in iron. People who are diagnosed with iron deficiency should consume red meat and increase other foods in the diet that are good sources of iron. This iron-rich diet should be implemented for at least three months and iron levels should be checked at the end of this period. If a desired level of iron isn't achieved through diet, supplements can be used to solve the problem. However, improved nutrition should always be the first solution attempted to solve such problems.

Zinc: Zinc is an element embedded into the structures of hundreds of enzymes and proteins. In women, zinc cooperates with more than 300 different enzymes to keep the body healthy. These enzymes, which have very important tasks, cannot function at sufficient levels when there is a zinc deficiency, and these problems extend to the reproductive system. Without zinc, your cells cannot self-divide properly; estrogen and progesterone levels can become imbalanced and your reproductive system can totally lose its function. According to the Supported Reproductive Technology reports of the U.S. Centers for Disease Control, low zinc levels are directly linked to miscarriages in the early stages of pregnancy.

Zinc is also considered to be one of the most important minerals for male fertility. Increasing zinc levels have been observed to increase sperm levels in men. Zinc also enhances sperm morphology, function and quality, while decreasing infertility.

Zinc is available in egg yolk, seeds, wheat and other grains.

Whole Grain Foods Grains are the main source of nourishment that constitute carbohydrates in our kitchen. Bread, pasta, and pastries are all classified as grain foods. This group forms the basis of our cuisine. "Unprocessed

whole grains" should be our choice in this food category. Whole-grain foods include all components of grains, namely the outside, middle and inner layers. The bran, or outer layer, is more resistant to digestion and slows down the digestive process. As a result, blood sugar increases more slowly and reproductive hormones are affected less.
Our body easily digests starch and gets it into our blood circulation. Digestion of fiber-rich foods takes more time because cellulose, which forms the fiber structure, cannot be easily digested by humans. Whole grains and vegetables that are in the group of fiber foods are very good for our body, because they require longer, more gradual digestion.

But what happens to the grain if it gets processed? Its outside protective fiber layer is removed, and its inner part, which is rich in nutrients, remains. Our body easily and quickly digests the nutrients in this processed form of the grain without encountering any obstacles, and this causes a spike in our blood sugar. The outer layer, besides having lots of fiber, is also full of vitamin B and iron. Throwing away this layer leads to a decrease in vitamin B and iron, which are very important for female reproduction. Opting for high-fiber products in the category of grain foods is one of the indispensables of the Motherhood Diet.

Suggested Resource*: If you would like to have comparative information at hand about the vitamin and mineral contents of food items in terms of nutrients, diet and components, the National Food Composition Database (Turkomp), available on the website of the Ministry of Food, Agriculture and Livestock, would be a very good source.*

On TurKomp, you can see data related to 63,000 nutrients and energy values for 100 food components belonging to 580 foods, from 14 food groups. Web address: www.turkomp.gov.tr

Pregnancy for Vegetarians and Vegans

A vegetarian or vegan diet is not an obstacle to a healthy pregnancy; however, one should take care of nutritional deficiencies that can show up in the body. Your body's needs for extra iron (can be measured via blood tests), folate (should be taken as a complementary supplement in any case), iodine, vitamin B12, vitamin D3, and zinc should be identified before and after conception. Additionally, those who do not consume dairy products have to ensure sufficient calcium intake through other foods. DHA, like Omega3, fatty acids and iodine supplements, is a recommended supplement for those who do not eat fish.

A plain vegan diet poses a risk for the mother and development of the baby. Improper nutrition could lead to a sad and irreversible outcome for your baby, such as a major impairment in the formation of the nervous system. If you are following a vegan diet, you need to have a detailed medical checkup and get certain complementary micronutrients, proteins and fats.

THE EFFECTS OF BEVERAGES ON FERTILITY

We tend to think more about solid foods, but drinks can have a high impact on our health and fertility. Therefore, I would like to touch upon this subject.

Caffeinated drinks: Caffeine, which is present in coffee, tea, cacao seeds, some herbal teas, and cola drinks, increases stress hormones, accelerates the pulse and stimulates the person by increasing adrenaline and dopamine secretion. The effect of caffeine on people varies, but if daily intake is around 150-200 milliliters, the person will usually experience some sleep problems. While caffeine is metabolized by 50% within six hours in a normal adult, this rate becomes 11 hours in pregnant women, and over 100 hours in the fetus, as adults have a metabolic process to deal with caffeine that has yet to form in the baby. The metabolism of the pregnant woman determines the rate at which caffeine transferred to the fetus. Two pregnant women may drink the same amount of coffee, but if their metabolic features are different, the amount of caffeine transferred to their babies will also vary. When you consume caffeine on a regular basis, your baby will face the risk of developmental delays. The research indicates that babies born to mothers who consume 200 milligrams of caffeine daily are born an average of 60–70 grams lighter. The same research also compared the weights of two groups of babies: ones born to mothers who consumed 300 milligrams of caffeine daily before conception and lowered it to 50 milligrams during pregnancy, and those born to mothers who kept their 300 milligrams of daily caffeine consumption after conception. At the end of the study, a lower weight of 150 grams was observed in the second group, the babies born to mothers who maintained their pre-pregnancy caffeine consumption during pregnancy.

The risk doubles when both alcohol and coffee are consumed by the mother. If you are trying to conceive, you need to refrain from caffeinated drinks, because women who drink three or more cups of coffee on a daily basis have a 15%–20% lower fertility rate around the time of ovulation. Exceeding this amount of caffeine may scuttle the fertility process altogether and cause miscarriages.

Caffeine content of certain kinds of coffee and tea:	Caffeine
1 cup of filtered coffee	135–200 mg
1 cup of espresso	100 mg
1 cup of cappuccino	100 mg
1 cup of Turkish coffee	57 mg
150 cc instant coffee	57 mg
150 cc decaffeinated coffee	5 mg
175 cc brewed tea	20–110 mg
330 cc iced tea	70 mg
200 cc teabag	30 mg
1 can of coke	30–56 mg
1 can of diet coke	38–45 mg
1 can of soda	Around 50 mg
1 can of fruit soda	0 mg
1 cup of tea	50 mg
1 can of energy drink	80 mg
50 grams of chocolate	50 mg
100 grams of milk chocolate	20 mg

Alcoholic drinks: An alcohol consumption of 7–8 glasses per week is known to reduce fertility in a definite way. Having even one glass of alcohol per week decreases the chance of getting pregnant in comparison to those who do not drink any. Alcohol impacts ovary function adversely and increases the risk of chromosome abnormalities in the baby. According to research, consuming 1–5 glasses of alcohol per week decreases the average fertility rate to 61%, while more than 10 glasses per week lowers it to 34%. Alcohol also increases the risk of miscarriage.

Carbonated beverages: Blood sugar increases within 20 minutes after consuming carbonated beverages, which contain harmful substances such as sweeteners, simple sugars, chemicals, colorants, and preservatives, and an insulin burst takes place right after. Due to an elevated hormone level, the liver rapidly turns the sugar into fat. People who consume carbonated beverages a lot have a higher probability of developing type 2 diabetes. These beverages also increase the risk of osteoporosis and bone breakage in the long run, in part because they contain phosphoric acid and high rates of phosphate. They can also pave the way for heart diseases, asthma, dental problems, and kidney diseases. Soda cans are covered with a kind of resin that has a high BPA content. This chemical, sometimes present in plastic and even baby bottles, is a cancer-causing substance that harms endocrine glands, and prompts the early onset of puberty and reproductive system disorders.

Mineral water: Mineral water is characterized as water that originates from underground sources and contains at least 250 milligrams of dissolved solids per liter. Water that contains less than 500 milligrams of mineral per liter is described as low-mineral water and water that contains more than 1500 milligrams per liter is described as high-mineral water. You should have a blood test to see which minerals are deficient in your body so as to make a healthy choice, as different brands on the market contain different amounts of minerals. A mineral water that is formed by merely adding carbon dioxide to any kind of water has no function other than relaxing the stomach.

A prospective mother's body needs food, liquids, minerals and vitamins that support fertility to nourish and grow a baby. If you are not experiencing heart, kidney and hypertension problems during this period, you can consume a bottle of mineral water daily in order to get a portion of the minerals your body needs. This not only prevents dehydration, but also offers a better alternative to sweet and carbonated beverages and even to regular tap water. The study published in the *International Journal of Laboratory Hematology* in 2003 states that mineral water is quite helpful in preventing iron deficiency in pregnancy. I recommend you consume glass-bottled mineral water and drink it from a glass cup rather than a plastic one.

Fruit Juice, Iced Tea, Compote and Khoshaf [5]**:** Off-the-shelf fruit juices and iced tea contain high amounts of sugar, and this is not something you need. Eating fruit is much more beneficial than drinking fruit juice. I can hear you asking what the most innocent drink would be if we want to drink something with a meal. If you are in the habit, I recommend preparing sugar-free compote and khoshaf for yourself. You may gradually decrease the sugar content of compote and khoshaf until they become sugar-free, to get used to the taste. Mixing various fruits rather than using fruits with high sugar content could be another alternative.

Orange juice is also effective in preventing certain birth defects for women who are pregnant or trying to get pregnant. As folic acid need increases during this period, a glass of orange juice can help meet folate and Vitamin C needs, provided that oranges are in season. However, one should cease taking orange juice as of the third month of pregnancy and replace it with pears and apples.

Herbal Teas: As you know, some medications are produced from herbs. Herbal teas, even if they are quite

[5] Dried fruit and nut compote

healthy, can change your hormonal balance. For this reason, your doctor or dietitian should decide the kind and amount of the tea that will be good for you by looking at your blood values, and you should follow their advice! For instance, there are some studies indicating that green tea diminishes the folic acid absorption that is necessary for fertility and a healthy pregnancy. If you want to consume herbal teas, first consider the effect they might have on you and enjoy them in a conscious way, according to what your body needs.

Milk and yoghurt drinks: Most of us are confused when it comes to milk. It is said that processed milk products are not very beneficial and may actually do more harm than good. On the other hand, the healthiness of unprocessed milk that has not been to any facility is questionable, as it does not undergo any kind of inspection. The wisest thing to do is to consume unskimmed dairy milk. Goat milk and almond milk are also good alternatives. Those with milk and yoghurt intolerance can meet their calcium needs from sources such as sesame, tofu, almond, flaxseed, cheese, and green-leafy vegetables.

Md. Colin Campbell, an American biochemist and author of *The China Study*, points out that casein, which forms 87% of the protein in cow's milk, encourages the progress of cancer. He also adds that milk consumption paves the way for cancer, as there is a high chance milk can be contaminated with aflatoxin[6]*, a highly carcinogenic substance. In his book, he claims that the calcium content of

---

[6] **Aflatoxin:** It is one of the carcinogenic chemicals produced by the molds we come across everywhere in our daily lives. In addition to affecting many organs, its direct or indirect ingestion especially increases the risk of liver cancer.

milk renders calcium absorption by the bones more difficult, contrary to strengthening them, and that osteoporosis is more commonly observed in societies consuming more milk.

Water: We all know how important water is for our body. If you are not sure whether you are drinking 1.5–2 liters of water every day, and if you forget to drink water, you may set an hourly reminder on your mobile device. Having a one-liter glass bottle by your computer or in your living room could serve as another reminder. Please take care not to use a plastic container for your water.

FERTILITY ENHANCING FOODS

Raspberry leaves: Raspberry leaves, which contain estrogen, help with optimizing egg maturation in the first half of the menstruation cycle. You can brew dried raspberry leaves the way you'd brew a pot of tea. Keep the leaves in cold water for 1–2 hours and boil them in the same water. One teaspoon of dried leaves is enough for a cup of raspberry tea.

Lady's mantle: Lady's mantle, which has been used to increase female fertility for centuries, has some features such as regulating menstrual cycles, strengthening uterus walls and increasing blood circulation. This herb, which has a very good anti-inflammatory[7] effect can also be consumed for progesterone[8]. When you consume this herb, which also eliminates premenstrual tension, pay attention to not brewing the tea any longer than ten minutes and consume it an hour after meals. Please consume it without mixing in sweeteners and other substances.

Avocado: Avocado increases energy levels with its high folic acid content. It may also boost male hormone production with its vitamin B6 and potassium. The ancient Aztecs, who linked the avocado tree with fertility, called it the "testicle tree." You can have ripe avocado on your breakfast plate or in your salads. You can consume this fruit, which is also said to create an aphrodisiac effect, together with your spouse three times in a week, because it supports fertility and increases sperm count.

---

[7]**Inflammatory:** Body's response to allergen, some sort of inflammation.
[8]**Progesterone:** A steroid hormone with 21 carbons that plays a role in the menstrual cycle, pregnancy and embryogenesis in humans and animals.

Sunflower seeds: Sunflower seeds support reproductive health in both sexes, with their rich zinc content. The selenium in these seeds promotes production of the progesterone hormone. However, you should be sure to eat them in small amounts due to their high calorie content.

Almonds: Almonds contain Omega6 fatty acids, vitamins E and B2, magnesium and calcium. While they help with testosterone production in men, they are also believed to create aphrodisiac effects in women. You can sprinkle almonds on your breakfast cereals, use them in your smoothies or turn them into almond milk as an alternative to cow's milk. The healthy unsaturated fat content of almonds increases fertility in women and also affects sperm production positively due to vitamin E.

Fish and oysters: As fish is a great source of vitamins and minerals, two servings of fatty fish per week increase the chances of getting pregnant. It is helpful to consume fatty fish such as mackerel, salmon, sardines, anchovy, menhaden and albacore once a week. As zinc deficiency slows down egg development, you may also include in your diet neatly cleaned oysters, which are rich in zinc. In a study conducted by Yale University, 63% of women who were unable to conceive were found to be vitamin D deficient. The most important vitamin D source is salmon.

Bulgur: Bulgur, an important source of carbohydrates, has a diverse content, including selenium, folic acid, vitamins B and B12, that supports fertility. It has a special place in this diet thanks to its ability to balance blood sugar.

Strawberry: Being full of antioxidants, it helps to delay aging, protect the egg from harm, and increase sperm count with its rich vitamin E content. It also increases sexual desire.

Basil: Even though basil is recognized as an herbal flavoring, it is also a medical herb that has considerable effects on the body. It contains estrogen-like compounds, and this helps with the maturation of the egg. Basil makes you feel good and improves the circulation. You can add its fresh leaves to salads, sandwiches, soups and sauces.

Carrot: Carrots, which are rich in vitamin A, can help regulate the menstrual cycle of women. They can also increase sperm quality, more so than other fruits and vegetables due to their carotenoid content. The antioxidants in carrot render ineffective free radicals that damage cell membranes and DNA.

Pumpkin seed: Pumpkin seeds increase testosterone production in men due to their high zinc and essential fatty acid content. They are rich in Omega3, which plays an important role in sexual health and is effective on prostaglandin production. They can be consumed in salads or smoothies.

Carob: Carob is a natural cholesterol- and fat-free dessert ingredient that is a good source of calcium, selenium and fiber. It meets 30% of the daily calcium requirement. It is good for intestinal health and enhances the activities of certain digestive enzymes. It is also functional in improving sperm count. Other positive features are its being antioxidant, antiseptic, antibacterial and anti-allergic. You can mix powdered carob into your yoghurt, use it as a natural dessert and consume it in the form of molasses.

Celery: Celery is a vegetable commonly consumed by those who would like to lose weight. It is rich in fiber and contains carbohydrates. It helps the body get rid of fluid retention and toxins. Celery is also a source of vitamins A and C, sodium, silicium, calcium, magnesium and iron. It increases the activity of white blood cells and supports pregnancy by means of an increase in blood volume. When consumed raw by men, it enables the secretion of pheromone (a chemical substance secreted externally) that attracts the opposite sex. It also has a healing effect on the mood.

Asparagus: Asparagus is rich in vitamin E. It is important for sleep and is said to arouse sexual desire. Its folic acid content plays a key role in the development of a healthy fetus.

Cabbage group: Cabbage, kale, and other cruciferous vegetables affect estrogen balance positively. Cabbage is an important source of folate (folic acid), contains vitamin C, and has antioxidant features. As a result, it helps to protect egg and sperm from free radicals. Broccoli, cauliflower and arugula have similar functions. It's helpful to consume them cooked, for better digestion and absorption.

Maca root: This plant, which grows in Peru, is known as natural Viagra. It increases sexual desire in both sexes and enhances sperm quantity, helps with erection problems in men, and increases fertility in women. It also raises energy levels with its vitamin, mineral and amino acid content. Small amounts are recommended in the initial stages of the diet. You can add a teaspoon of powdered maca root to your smoothies.

Lentil: A scientific study carried out by Harvard University proves the importance of vegetable protein and iron in terms of fertility. The fertility rates of women who consume vegetable protein and iron increase by 30%. A cup of cooked lentils, which are rich in folic acid, iron, fiber and protein, is enough to meet the daily folic acid need by 90%.

Banana: Banana, being a good source of B group vitamins and potassium, supports the production of estrogen and testosterone in women and men, respectively. Best consumed raw, banana increases energy levels thanks to its vitamin B content and is also said to increase sexual desire in men.

Absinthe plant: It helps to regulate hormonal levels in women with irregular menstrual cycles. Absinthe stimulates hormone production and supports the maturation of the oocyte (egg).

Garlic: Garlic is very good for the immune system and contains allicin, which increases blood flow to the sexual organs. Its vitamin B and selenium content supports fertility. It is best consumed either raw or stewed, so that its extract blends into the dishes. You can also add crushed garlic to sauces or spreads.

NUTRITION ON SPECIAL DAYS

In every culture, desserts are consumed at birthdays, celebrations, holiday seasons and special times such as Ramadan, Christmas and Hanukah. When we visit another household or have guests at home, treats are usually more abundant than what we normally eat. In such cases, you should try to keep up with your diet as much as possible and request your social circle not to ask you to indulge in the treats, by letting them know that you are on a diet for a special reason. Your family and friends are very likely to be understanding, but if they still insist, just take very limited portions on your plate, mostly from the harmless options, and try to consume only half of that! By doing so, you can pull through the special times with the least harm.

Desserts with sherbet or syrup are digested very quickly by the body, making the blood sugar surge. It is better for the regulation of blood sugar to consume bitter chocolate instead of syrup or sherbet desserts. If you crave something to complement your tea after the meal, fresh walnuts, almonds, or hazelnuts would be a much better choice than desserts.

Pay special attention to the content of the Iftar dinner during Ramadan, to be sure the food you're eating doesn't include simple carbohydrates and sugars. Refrain from eating food such as rice, pasta and pastries at Iftar and Sahur.

Ramadan meals should mostly concentrate on the following;

1. Proteins
2. Carbohydrates from fibrous vegetables such as spinach and artichoke
3. Avoid pasta, bread, rice
4. Avoid consuming large amounts of food
5. Avoid dessert after the meal

Instead of rice pilaf, try to consume carbohydrate sources that are digested more slowly, such as beans, chickpeas, lentils, leeks and spinach. Do not eat bread with your meal, and if you can't help this, opt for whole grains or whole-wheat bread.

HOW TO DO A FERTILITY DETOX

Over the course of years, our bodies accumulate toxins from air, soil, water, electromagnetic waves, and chemicals that are present in the products we consume daily. The majority of these toxins are stored in the fat tissues of the body and can only be eliminated from the body through cleansing. Alcohol, smoking, excessive hormones, improper nutrition, pesticides (in the vegetables and fruits we consume) and hormonal birth control methods constitute only a few of the ways toxins enter our body.

We need to purify ourselves from these toxins to have a healthy body. Detox is a method that has been used to accomplish this for thousands of years, in all corners of the world. This purification may be one of the most useful things that can be done prior to pregnancy, and to keep the body healthy in a natural way. Fertility detox supports the body by cleansing the uterus and liver of excessive toxins and hormones. It cleans the uterus of dirty blood as well as strengthening the uterus and increasing blood circulation.

Detox should not be implemented during pregnancy or breastfeeding. As this process purifies your body of toxins, your baby will be subjected to these substances and s/he can be harmed. People suffering from hypertension, blood sugar disorders, diabetes and anemia, and those working at jobs requiring strenuous physical activity or taking pills on a regular basis also should not do detox. Even though any kind of detox helps purify the body, the "fertility detox," which aims to support functions of the reproductive system and eliminate substances that harm fertility, concentrates on the liver and uterus.

Liver: The liver is the organ that helps us filter toxins, including excessive hormones, out of our bodies. If there is an estrogen surplus in your body, it is the task of liver to get rid of it. Malnutrition, lifestyle, and general health problems necessitate the stimulation of the liver. If you would like your body to remain more resistant to an industrial world, you can benefit from certain herbs and plants that I will talk about soon.

Uterus: The health of the uterus is extremely important for reproduction. The tissue structure and environment of the uterus have been formed for the embryo. As you might guess, a healthy environment will not be formed for the embryo if old stagnant blood remains in the womb and toxins accumulate therein during each menstrual bleeding. The reasons for toxin accumulation might include low circulation, hormonal imbalance and unhealthy diet. The herbs that I will talk about support your blood circulation, regulate the circulation in the uterus, and strengthen the muscles; in summary, they support the formation of a healthy uterine environment.

The uterus needs proper circulation to carry out its function in the best way: balanced blood circulation between the womb and ovaries, which must work smoothly with the endocrine system. Circulation necessary for proper hormonal balance will increase hormone production while protecting the menstrual cycle. Exercise, plants and massage can be other effective ways to gain benefits in terms of circulation.

Cleansing herbs for fertility

For the liver:

- Greater burdock (Arctium lappa)
- Milk thistle extract
- Sow thistle extract
- Dandelion herb
- Yellow dock root
- Licorice root
- Ginger

Herbs that cleanse and tone the uterus

-Goldenseal

-Dong quai root

-Peony root

-Raspberry leaves

How to do the detox:

• The objective of detoxing is to relax the digestive system, because in your daily routine, the body spends a great deal of time and energy accomplishing digestion. Digestion of a meat dish takes about 6–8 hours, while a carbohydrate dish is digested in 3–4 hours. This period is about 1–2 hours for a vegetable dish and half an hour for fruits.

• Consume a large bowl of salad every single day. Fibrous foods clean the body of excessive hormones and enable you to get necessary minerals. Only one meal should be solid, and the rest should be liquid during the day.

• You can detox during seasonal transitions. You can do the detox for 5–7 days if you get solid food in one meal per day. If you are planning to feed on liquids for three meals, then three days of detoxing will be sufficient. Using the single solid meal approach, you can consume a smoothie, green juice or soup at breakfast and dinner and have solid food at lunch. It will be more functional to have your solid food at lunchtime, when your metabolism is at the highest energy level.

• You can consume vegetables, herbs, brown rice, gluten-free grains, stevia, beans, lentils, green tea, fish, organic chicken or turkey, nuts, seeds, avocado, coconut and fruits as solid food. Please do not choose milk products, gluten, processed sugar, coffee, sodas, alcohol, corn, tomatoes, eggplant, peppers, bananas, strawberry, oranges or grapes. Last but not least, do not consume any harmful foods or beverages, such as deli products and alcohol!

• You can use the recommended herbs and plants in your smoothies.

• If you are planning to have two solid meals, there should be a minimum 12 hours in between those meals, for allowing the detox process to fulfill its function. The body completes digestion and starts the detox signal in the eighth hour and completes the detox in the twelfth hour. For example, if you had your dinner at 7 p.m., your next meal should be at 7 a.m. at the earliest.

• You can repeat this every season, and I recommend you detox at least twice a year.

Sample recipe

Liver-friendly juice
300 milliliters of water
2 large grapefruits
2 tablespoons of flaxseed oil
4 lemons
5 centimeters of fresh ginger root
1 clove of garlic

Preparation

Squeeze the lemons and grapefruits. Crush the garlic and ginger, add them to the juice and mix them in blender. Add the flaxseed oil, two probiotic capsules and water. Blend them for 4–5 seconds.

Benefits:

This recipe contributes to your detox by helping the liver cleanse itself.

Mealtime: LUNCH or DINNER

Note: For best results, do not have tea or coffee when you drink this juice, and consume a lot of water. **Seasons:** Fall, winter, spring

While detoxing;

1. Daily toxin discharge: The easiest way of doing this is to drink water with lemon right after you wake up. Squeezing half a lemon into 1 liter of water is sufficient. This will help clean your liver. Besides, the vitamin C and antioxidant content of lemon is effective in terms of maintaining your hormonal balance.

2. Move: Our body has been designed to move, not to sit still. Every single breath we take while exercising provides us with oxygen and muscle relaxation, and these all lower stress. It will be beneficial to choose less-intensive sports such as dance, yoga or walking. Light movements enable you to get rid of toxins more easily. Intensive sports are not recommended during detox, as they cause the accumulation of lactic acid in the body.

3. Fertility diet: Your diet, which consists of very healthy foods, will be your best helper in flushing toxins from the body.

4. Brush and rub your body with a coarse bath-glove: Your skin is the largest organ of your body, and one third of toxins are discharged from body through the skin. For this reason, brushing and rubbing your skin with a coarse bath-glove is not only effective for toxin removal but also contributes to the lymphatic system's performance. Energizing the body and treating cellulite are other benefits. It is beneficial to brush in an upward direction. Visiting a steam room or sauna is also one of the most important parts of a detox program. Toxins that accumulate in the lymphatic system can be easily expelled from the body by taking a steam bath. It is also very good for weight loss, fatty liver syndrome, treating the aches and pains in the body, and beautification of the skin. It is possible to perspire at a much lower temperature in infrared saunas.

5. Fertility massage: Different kinds of massage lead to removal of toxins from the body by triggering a movement in the lymphatic system. Stomach massage is most efficacious for those who have a constipation problem. Reflexology can support fertility massage. Rub your big toes with circular movements and then give a fertility massage to your uterus area.

6. Keep away from chemicals and radiation: If possible, keep away from mobile phone devices and base stations. Take a short vacation somewhere without mobile phone reception, like Mount Ida in Turkey, for instance. Try to use organic materials if you apply makeup, and pick cleaning products that do not have harmful chemicals.

FERTILITY MASSAGE

The fountainhead of fertility massage, which is considered one of the best treatments abroad, has the goal of helping the reproductive system by increasing blood flow, maintaining hormonal balance and purifying the body of toxins. A massage is applied on the ovaries and uterus in this method, which is usually recommended in the course of IVF treatments to enable the embryo to get a better grip on the uterus.

It is important to apply circular massages in the belly and pelvic region using both hands. When this massage is done regularly, it increases the chance of pregnancy by boosting blood supply to the ovaries and uterus.

You can turn this massage into a habit right before you get up from bed or right after your daily exercise. The healthiest option would be to do it every other day. This massage, which you should not do during your menstrual bleeding, may not only increase fertility but also help prevent ovarian cysts. Start the massage when your menstrual period ends and keep doing it until the end of ovulation. You can do the massage yourself or ask your spouse to do it for you.

Relax your mind during this massage, which will serve as therapy for you. Just focus on your baby and health. Start your day in a positive mood, thinking about nice things.

How to perform a fertility massage:

1. If you wish, put a little massage oil on your abdomen. Position your hands on both sides of your navel, breathe calmly and deeply. Then massage your abdomen and uterus in clockwise circles that are the size of a large orange.

2. Massage on your big toes, which form one of the acupuncture points, is very effective as well. Apply pressure on your big toes by making small clockwise circles.

3. Massage your abdomen, starting from the intersection point of your breasts to your vagina, pressing with both hands and using four fingers in each hand, and in the form of two parallel lines. In the same way, continue the massage by putting your hands on the point where your vagina starts and apply pressure with four fingers toward your navel. Stop massaging during your menstrual bleeding or pregnancy. The effectiveness of massage is relevant to your implementation of the fertility diet. As this diet has a nutritional content that increases blood flow, you will gain maximum benefit from massage when you support it with the diet.

4. Slightly press your womb and navel area while massaging. Apply pressure in a way that will not hurt you. Your hand movements should be absolutely circular when you apply the massage. You need to massage the right and left ovaries separately. The massage that will start right below your ribcage and move in the direction of your ovaries should last 15 minutes daily. You should wait at least 1.5–2 hours to do it after meals.

Benefits of Massage:

- Drives blood out of the body.
- Prevents menstrual cramps and regulates your menstrual cycles. Regulates endocrine system.
- Increases and accelerates blood flow to the reproductive organs.
- Reduces stress.
- Balances hormones.

SAMPLE DIET THAT WILL INCREASE YOUR FERTILITY

It is recommended that your daily energy intake be no less than 1800 calories per day during the pre-pregnancy and pregnancy periods. For this reason, we have arranged the energy content of sample menus based on an 1800-calorie diet plan. This diet was prepared based on people within the 30–35 age range, at a normal weight and with normal blood values.

If you primarily have to lose or gain weight to increase your fertility and have a healthy pregnancy, it will be more beneficial for you to initially follow another diet prepared by your dietitian and then move on to this diet.

It's important to consume all the food items on the menu for adequate and balanced nutrition. Also, please keep the following in mind while implementing this diet:

1. You need to drink at least 8–10 glasses of water per day.

2. You can drink herbal teas such as green tea, linden tea, rose hip tea, apple tea and other fruit teas, but you should limit your daily consumption to two cups and brew the tea for 3–4 minutes.

3. Pay attention to consuming fruits and vegetables that are naturally in season and grown organically without the use of pesticides.

4. Use olive oil in your dishes, taking care not to burn the oil while cooking.

5. Use onion and garlic abundantly while cooking.

6. Use fat-free bone broth to enhance the nutritional values of soups and dishes.

7. Limit your daily salt consumption to 5 grams and use iodized salt.

8. Pay attention to regular mealtimes and having your breakfast within half an hour of waking up if you are on a thyroid hormone pill.

9. Have your night snack two hours before you go to bed.

10. Do not consume caffeinated drinks such as strong tea, coffee, cola, and alcoholic drinks.

11. Avoid sugar or artificial sweeteners.

12. Do not consume processed foods (off-the-shelf packaged products).

How to calculate your daily calorie needs

Daily calorie needs vary from one person to another. At this point, the most important factor is that the amount of food consumed should be equivalent to the energy burned during your daily activities, in addition to the basal metabolic rate calculated by using weight, height, and age of the person. The following is the formula to calculate the basal metabolic rate:

Basal metabolic rate in women:
655 + 9.6 X (weight in kilograms) + 1.8 X (height in centimeters) – 4.7 X (age)
Basal metabolic rate in men:
66 + 13.7 X (weight in kilograms) + 5 X (height in centimeters) – 6.8 X (age)

7-DAY FALL MENU

DAY 1

BREAKFAST

1 cup of weak tea

Toasted sandwich with cheddar cheese (2 thin slices of sour whole rye bread with a layer of cheddar cheese slices–60 grams)

1 medium-size clementine

SNACK

1 glass of water, 1 medium size kiwi

LUNCH

1 serving of meatball soup with egg yolk and lemon sauce

1 bowl of basil carrot salad with a bit of oil

1 thin slice of whole-wheat sourdough bread

MID-AFTERNOON

10 fresh almonds and 2 damson plums

DINNER

1 bowl of cabbage soup

6 tablespoons of black-eyed beans with olive oil

1 bowl of yoghurt with walnuts

SNACK

1 glass of kefir and two whole raw walnuts

Total calories 1798 (kcal)

DAY 2

BREAKFAST

1 glass of milk

1 boiled egg

1 slice of (30 grams) dil cheese (a kind of cheese similar to unsalted mozzarella)

2 whole raw walnuts

1 medium size tomato, 1 medium size cucumber, 2–3 green peppers

1 thin slice of whole wheat sourdough bread

SNACK

10 fresh hazelnuts and 1 medium-size pear

LUNCH

6 tablespoons of eggplant dish prepared using olive oil

1 bowl of avocado salad

1 glass of kefir

1 thin slice of whole-wheat sourdough bread

MID-AFTERNOON

1 bowl of yoghurt with half a banana and two tablespoons of pomegranate seeds

DINNER

1 serving of anchovy (150 grams or 5.3 ounces)

1 bowl of seasonal salad with a dash of olive oil

SNACK

1 handful of roasted chickpeas and 15 raisins

Total calories 1821 (kcal)

DAY 3

BREAKFAST
1 glass of kefir mixed with 3 tablespoons of oatmeal, 10 fresh almonds
1 slice of pineapple, 1 medium-size fig

SNACK
1 bowl of blueberries

LUNCH
1 serving of sautéed chicken
3 tablespoons of bulgur pilaf mixed with green lentils
1 bowl of tzatziki

MID-AFTERNOON
2 carobs and 2 handfuls of sunflower seeds

DINNER
1 bowl of tarhana soup
6 tablespoons of zucchini stew cooked with ground beef
1 bowl of yoghurt
1 thin slice of sour whole rye bread

SNACK
1 medium size apple

Total calories 1780 (kcal)

DAY 4

BREAKFAST

1 cup of weak tea

1 serving of scrambled eggs with chopped tomatoes and sliced green peppers

(ingredients: 1 egg, 1 medium-size tomato, 2–3 green peppers, 1 teaspoon of olive oil)

1 slice of (30 grams) feta cheese

3–4 black olives

1 thin slice of whole-wheat sourdough bread

SNACK

1 glass of milk and 15 black grapes

LUNCH

6 tablespoons of stew with okra and chickpeas

1 bowl of roasted red peppers with yoghurt

1 thin slice of whole-wheat sourdough bread

MID-AFTERNOON

A slice of watermelon about 2 inches thick

DINNER

1 serving of green salad with avocados and grilled steak (150 grams of grilled steak, half avocado, 2 whole raw walnuts, lettuce, arugula, basil, parsley, dill, 1 tablespoon of olive oil)

1 glass of kefir

SNACK

10 raw hazelnuts and 1 medium size kiwi

Total calories 1815 (kcal)

DAY 5

BREAKFAST

1 glass of milk
2 slices of goat cheese (60 grams)
5–6 green olives
1 medium-size tomato, 1 medium-size cucumber, 2–3 green peppers
2 thin slices of sourdough whole rye bread

SNACK

1 slice of pineapple and 2 handfuls of pumpkin seeds

LUNCH

1 serving of mackerel stew (150 grams)
1 bowl of arugula salad with walnuts and a dash of oil

MID-AFTERNOON

1 glass of kefir and 1 medium-size clementine

DINNER

1 bowl of lentil soup
6 tablespoons of spinach stew prepared using olive oil
1 bowl of yoghurt
1 thin slice of sourdough whole rye bread

SNACK

1 small pomegranate

Total calories 1795 (kcal)

DAY 6

BREAKFAST

1 cup of weak tea

2 slices of bread with pureed avocadoes and almonds (half of a medium avocado, 5–6 almonds, basil, parsley, dill, 1 tablespoon of olive oil, 2 thin slices of sourdough whole-wheat bread)

2 damson plums

SNACK

1 glass of milk and half of a medium-size quince

LUNCH

6 tablespoons of leeks cooked with eggs

1 bowl of carrot salad with a dash of oil

1 thin slice of sourdough whole-wheat bread

MID-AFTERNOON

2 whole raw walnuts and 2 carobs

DINNER

6 tablespoons of haricot bean stew with ground beef

3 tablespoons of bulgur pilaf with vegetables

1 bowl of shepherd's salad with a dash of oil

1 glass of yoghurt drink

SNACK

1 glass of kefir and half a cup of berries

Total calories 1818 (kcal)

DAY 7

BREAKFAST

1 glass of milk mixed with 3 spoons of oatmeal, 2 whole raw walnuts, half banana, 3 dried apricots

SNACK

A slice of watermelon about 2 inches thick and one slice of feta cheese (30 grams)

LUNCH

1 bowl of pumpkin soup
1 serving of cauliflower au gratin
1 bowl of lettuce salad with a dash of oil

MID-AFTERNOON

1 glass of kefir and 1 handful of white chickpeas

DINNER

1 serving of grilled bluefish (150 grams)
1 bowl of steamed broccoli with a dash of (1 tablespoon) olive oil

SNACK

10 raw hazelnuts and 1 medium size apple

Total calories 1803 (kcal)

7-DAY WINTER MENU

DAY 1

BREAKFAST

1 glass of milk with 3 tablespoons of oatmeal, 2 whole raw walnuts, 2 tablespoons of pomegranate, 1 tablespoon of dried black raisins

SNACK

1 medium-size apple

LUNCH

1 bowl of red lentil soup

6 tablespoons of celery stew prepared with orange juice

1 bowl of yoghurt

1 thin slice of sourdough whole-wheat bread

MID-AFTERNOON

Half of a medium-size quince and 10 raw hazelnuts

DINNER

1 serving of grilled mackerel

1 bowl of steamed mixed winter vegetables with 1 tablespoon of olive oil (brussels sprouts, carrots, cauliflower)

1 thin slice of sourdough whole rye bread

SNACK

1 glass of kefir and 10 raw almonds

Total calories 1815 (kcal)

DAY 2

BREAKFAST

1 glass of milk
1 boiled egg
2 tablespoons of whey cheese
5–6 green olives
Parsley-dill
2 thin slices of sourdough whole-wheat bread

SNACK

1 medium-size orange and 10 raw almonds

LUNCH

6 tablespoons of chickpeas with lamb meat
3 tablespoons of bulgur pilaf with vegetables
1 bowl of carrot salad with beets and a dash of oil

MID-AFTERNOON

1 glass of kefir and 5 dried plums

DINNER

6 tablespoons of leek stew prepared using olive oil
1 bowl of yoghurt avocado salad
1 thin slice of whole-wheat sourdough bread

SNACK

1 small pomegranate

Total calories 1798 (kcal)

DAY 3

BREAKFAST

1 cup of weak tea

Toasted sandwich with goat cheese (2 thin slices of sour rye bread with a layer of goat cheese slices–60 grams)

3 dried apricots, 2 whole raw walnuts

SNACK

1 glass of kefir and 1 medium-size kiwi

LUNCH

1 serving of oven-grilled salmon with vegetables (150 grams)

1 bowl of arugula salad with a zest of oil

1 thin slice of sour rye bread

MID-AFTERNOON

1 small winter pear and 1 medium-size clementine

DINNER

1 bowl of tarhana soup

6 tablespoons of cauliflower ground-beef stew

1 glass of yoghurt drink (ayran)

SNACK

1 glass of milk and 10 raw hazelnuts

Total calories 1783 (kcal)

DAY 4

BREAKFAST

1 cup of weak tea

2 slices of bread baked with eggs (1 egg, 30 grams of kashar cheese, parsley, dill, 1 teaspoon of olive oil, 2 thin slices of sour whole rye bread)

1 medium-size clementine

SNACK

1 small pomegranate

LUNCH

1 bowl of ezogelin soup

1 serving of spinach salad with tulum cheese (similar to bryndza) and walnuts (50 grams of tulum cheese, 2 whole walnuts, half a small bunch of spinach, 1 tablespoon of olive oil)

1 thin slice of sour whole-wheat bread

MID-AFTERNOON

1 glass of milk and 10 raw almonds

DINNER

1 serving of baked chicken thighs (150 grams)

1 bowl of steamed broccoli with one tablespoon of olive oil

1 bowl of celery salad with yoghurt

SNACK

1 espresso cup of dried blueberries

Total calories 1821 (kcal)

DAY 5

BREAKFAST

1 glass of kefir mixed with 3 tablespoons of oatmeal, 10 raw almonds, 1 small grated apple

SNACK

1 medium-size orange

LUNCH

4 grilled meatballs

3 tablespoons of bulgur pilaf

1 bowl of avocado salad with lots of lemon juice

1 glass of yoghurt drink (ayran)

MID-AFTERNOON

10 raw hazelnuts and 3 dried apricots

DINNER

1 bowl of vegetable soup

6 tablespoons of dried shell beans with olive oil

1 bowl of yoghurt

SNACK

1 large winter pear

Total calories 1816 (kcal)

DAY 6

BREAKFAST

1 glass of milk

2 slices of (60 grams) feta cheese

5–6 black olives

Parsley and dill

2 thin slices of sour whole-wheat bread

SNACK

1 medium-size apple and 10 raw hazelnuts

LUNCH

6 tablespoons of chard sautéed with eggs

1 bowl of yoghurt

1 thin slice of sour whole-wheat bread

MID-AFTERNOON

1 espresso-cup of dried blueberry and 3 whole walnuts

DINNER

1 serving of poached anchovies (150 grams)

1 bowl of seasonal salad with a dash of oil

SNACK

1 glass of kefir and 1 small pomegranate

Total calories 1788 (kcal)

DAY 7

BREAKFAST

1 cup of weak tea

Cheese omelet (1 egg, 1 slice (30 grams) feta cheese, 1 tablespoon of olive oil)

5–6 green olives

1 medium-size clementine

1 thin slice of sour whole rye bread

SNACK

1 glass of kefir and 5 dried prunes

LUNCH

1 bowl of broccoli soup

8 tablespoons of green lentil salad with pomegranates and walnuts (2 tablespoons of pomegranates, 2 whole walnuts, parsley, dill, scallions, 1 tablespoon of olive oil)

MID-AFTERNOON

1 medium-size orange and half medium-size quince

DINNER

8 medium-size stuffed cabbage leaves (stuffed with meat and bulgur)

1 bowl of beet and carrot salad with a dash of oil

1 bowl of yoghurt

SNACK

1 medium-size kiwi and 10 raw almonds

Total calories 1799 (kcal)

7-DAY SPRING MENU

DAY 1

BREAKFAST
1 glass of milk
1 boiled egg
1 slice (30 grams) feta cheese
5–6 green olives
3 dried apricots
2 thin slices of sour whole-wheat bread

SNACK
1 medium-size apple and 10 raw peanuts

LUNCH
6 tablespoons of pea stew cooked with meat
3 tablespoons of bulgur pilaf
1 bowl of tzatziki

MID-AFTERNOON
1 glass of kefir and 12 strawberries

DINNER
1 bowl of vegetable soup
6 tablespoons of haricot beans cooked with olive oil
1 bowl of seasonal salad with a dash of oil

SNACK
1 bowl of mulberries and 2 whole walnuts

Total calories 1785 (kcal)

DAY 2

BREAKFAST

1 glass of kefir mixed with 3 tablespoons of oatmeal
2 whole walnuts
6 strawberries,
1 tablespoon of dried black currants with seeds

SNACK

5 greengages and 6 loquats

LUNCH

1 serving of oven-baked red mullet (150 grams)
1 bowl of arugula salad with a dash of oil
1 thin slice of sour whole-wheat bread

MID-AFTERNOON

10 raw hazelnuts and 1 handful of yellow chickpeas

DINNER

1 bowl of red lentil soup
2 slices of oven-baked zucchini patties
1 bowl of yoghurt

SNACK

1 glass of milk and 12 strawberries

Total calories 1799 (kcal)

DAY 3

BREAKFAST

1 cup of weak tea

Toasted sandwich with mozzarella string cheese (2 slices or 60 grams of cheese, 2 thin slices of sour whole-wheat bread)

3 dried apricots, 2 whole walnuts

SNACK

1 glass of kefir and 1 espresso-cup of dried blueberries

LUNCH

1 bowl of black-eyed bean soup

6 tablespoons of spinach with ground beef

1 bowl of yoghurt

MID-AFTERNOON

1 bowl of mulberries and 10 raw almonds

DINNER

1 serving of chicken shish (150 gram)

1 serving of asparagus salad with a dash of oil

1 glass of yoghurt drink (ayran)

SNACK

1 medium-size apple

Total calories 1780 (kcal)

DAY 4

BREAKFAST

1 glass of milk

Egg with whey cheese (1 egg, 2 tablespoons whey cheese, parsley, dill, 1 tablespoon olive oil)

5–6 black olives

1 thin slice of sour whole-wheat bread

SNACK

10 raw hazelnuts and 5 greengages

LUNCH

1 serving of grilled sirloin (150 grams)

1 bowl of green salad with avocado

MID-AFTERNOON

1 glass of kefir and 1 tablespoon of dried black currants with seeds

DINNER

1 bowl of tarhana soup with chickpeas

2 artichokes cooked with olive oil

1 thin slice of sour whole-wheat bread

SNACK

12 strawberries and 2 whole walnuts

Total calories 1813 (kcal)

DAY 5

BREAKFAST
1 glass of milk mixed with 3 tablespoons of oatmeal,
10 raw almonds,
3 dried apricots, 1 dried fig

SNACK
1 bowl of mulberries

LUNCH
6 tablespoons of fresh kidney beans with olive oil
1 bowl of purslane with yoghurt

MID-AFTERNOON
10 raw pistachios and 6 loquats

DINNER
1 serving of poached sea bass (150 grams)
1 bowl of arugula salad with walnuts
1 thin slice of sour whole-wheat bread

SNACK
1 glass of kefir and a handful of white chickpeas

Total calories 1798 (kcal)

DAY 6

BREAKFAST

1 cup of weak tea

1 boiled egg

2 slices of (60 grams) tulum cheese (similar to bryndza)

5–6 green olives

Parsley and dill

2 thin slices of sour whole-wheat bread

SNACK

1 glass of kefir and 10 raw almonds

LUNCH

1 bowl of red beet soup

2 stuffed zucchinis (stuffed with bulgur and ground beef)

1 bowl of yoghurt

MID-AFTERNOON

1 medium-size apple

DINNER

8 tablespoons of green lentil dish

1 bowl of carrot and turnip salad with a dash of oil

1 glass of yoghurt drink (ayran)

SNACK

12 strawberries and 5 greengages

Total calories 1793 (kcal)

DAY 7

BREAKFAST

1 cup of weak tea

2 slices of bread with pureed avocado and cheese (half avocado, 2 whole walnuts, 30 grams feta cheese, parsley, dill, 1 teaspoon olive oil, 2 thin slices sour whole rye bread)

SNACK

6 loquats

LUNCH

4 oven baked meatballs

3 tablespoons of bulgur with vegetables

1 bowl of steamed broccoli with a tablespoon of olive oil

MID-AFTERNOON

1 glass of kefir and 1 espresso-cup of dried blueberries

DINNER

1 bowl of ezogelin soup

6 tablespoons of broad beans with olive oil

1 bowl of yoghurt

1 thin slice of sour whole wheat bread

SNACK

1 bowl of mulberries and 10 raw hazelnuts

Total calories 1793 (kcal)

7-DAY SUMMER MENU

DAY 1

BREAKFAST

1 cup of weak tea

1 serving of eggs scrambled with tomatoes and green pepper (1 egg, 1 medium-size tomato, 2–3 green peppers, 1 tablespoon olive oil)

1 slice (30 grams) feta cheese

3 apricots

1 thin slice sour whole-wheat bread

SNACK

1 glass of milk and 10 raw hazelnuts

LUNCH

1 serving grilled salmon (150 grams)

4–5 steamed asparagus spears

1 bowl of arugula salad with tomatoes and olive oil

MID-AFTERNOON

1 handful of white chickpeas and 5 greengages

DINNER

6 tablespoons of sautéed chard with olive oil

1 bowl of avocado salad with yoghurt

1 thin slice of sour whole-wheat bread

SNACK

1 glass of kefir and 12 strawberries

Total calories 1826 (kcal)

DAY 2

BREAKFAST

1 glass of milk mixed with 3 tablespoons of oatmeal, 2 whole walnuts, 12 berries

SNACK

1 bowl of mulberries and 2 carobs

LUNCH

1 bowl of yoghurt soup with wheat and chickpeas
6 tablespoons of green beans with olive oil
1 thin slice of sour whole rye bread

MID-AFTERNOON

A slice of watermelon about 2 inches thick and 1 slice (30 grams) feta cheese

DINNER

1 serving of chicken salad with almonds (150 grams of grilled chicken breast, 10 raw almonds, arugula, lettuce, basil, red pepper, 1 teaspoon of olive oil)
1 glass of kefir

SNACK

1 medium-size peach and 2 handfuls of sunflower seeds

Total calories 1810 (kcal)

DAY 3

BREAKFAST

1 cup of weak tea

1 boiled egg

2 slices of bread with pureed avocado (half of a medium-size avocado, 2 whole walnuts, basil, parsley, dill, 1 teaspoon olive oil, 2 thin slices sour whole rye bread)

SNACK

1 glass of kefir and 2 damson plums

LUNCH

1 oven-baked split eggplant[1] *with meat filling (prepared without frying)*

3 tablespoons of bulgur pilaf

1 bowl of tzatziki

MID-AFTERNOON

10 raw hazelnuts and 12 cherries

DINNER

6 tablespoons of vegetable stew with olive oil

6 tablespoons of haricot beans salad with tahini

1 thin slice of sour whole rye bread

SNACK

1 bowl of yoghurt mixed with an espresso-cup of dried blueberries, and 3 apricots

Total calories 1788 (kcal)

DAY 4

BREAKFAST

1 cup of weak tea

Toasted sandwich with tomato, basil, goat cheese (2 slices or 60 grams), 2 slices of tomato

2–3 leaves of basil, 2 thin slices of sour whole wheat bread

5–6 black olives

SNACK

1 glass of milk and 1 bowl of black mulberries

LUNCH

1 bowl of green lentil soup

2 artichokes with olive oil

1 thin slice of sour whole-wheat bread

MID-AFTERNOON

1 glass of kefir and 10 raw peanuts

DINNER

1 serving of oven-baked sea bass with vegetables (150 grams)

1 bowl of cow pea salad

SNACK

A slice of melon about 2 inches thick and 1 slice (30 grams) feta cheese

Total calories 1820 (kcal)

DAY 5

BREAKFAST

1 glass of milk
1 boiled egg
2 tablespoons of whey cheese
2 whole walnuts
1 medium-size tomato, 1 medium-size cucumber, 2–3 green peppers
2 thin slices of sour whole rye bread

SNACK

10 raw hazelnuts and 5 greengages

LUNCH

6 tablespoons of okra with meat
3 tablespoons of bulgur pilaf
1 glass of kefir

MID-AFTERNOON

1 bowl of fruit salad with avocado (half an avocado, 7 cherries, 7 black grapes, 2 apricots)

DINNER

1 bowl of tomato soup
6 tablespoons of peas with olive oil
1 bowl of roasted eggplant with yoghurt

SNACK

1 medium-size peach and 1 handful of white chickpeas

Total calories 1804 (kcal)

DAY 6

BREAKFAST

1 glass of kefir mixed with 3 tablespoons of oatmeal, 10 raw almonds, 6 strawberries, 1 tablespoon of dried black currants with seeds

SNACK

A slice of watermelon about 2 inches thick

LUNCH

6 tablespoons of red shell beans with olive oil
1 bowl of zucchini salad with walnuts and a dash of oil
1 thin slice of sour whole-wheat bread

MID-AFTERNOON

2 handfuls of pumpkin seeds and 6 loquats

DINNER

8 medium-size stuffed grape leaves (stuffed with bulgur and ground beef)
1 bowl of shepherd's salad with a dash of oil
1 bowl of yoghurt

SNACK

1 glass of milk and 2 damson plums

Total calories 1780 (kcal)

DAY 7

BREAKFAST

1 glass of milk

2 slices (60 grams) feta cheese

5–6 green olives

1 medium-size tomato, 1 medium-size cucumber, 2–3 green peppers

2 thin slices of sour whole-wheat bread

SNACK

2 medium-size figs and 2 whole walnuts

LUNCH

1 bowl of tarhana soup

6 tablespoons purslane with ground beef

1 bowl of yoghurt

1 thin slice of sour whole-wheat bread

MID-AFTERNOON

2 carobs and 12 cherries

DINNER

6 tablespoons of chickpeas with olive oil

1 bowl of green salad with wheat

SNACK

1 glass of kefir and 10 raw hazelnuts

Total calories 1785 (kcal)

Chapter Four

MALE FACTOR & MALE FERTILITY

You should not think solely about female fertility when you hear the term *fertility*. While 15% to 20% of couples experience fertility problems, half of these problems stem from men. Just like women, men are also affected by outside factors such as unhealthy nutrition, stress, pollution and radiation; and they may have problems like low-quality sperm production and low sperm quantity and motility, due to health issues. It seems men must also get ready for this journey, both mentally and physically, for a higher quality of sperm production.

Let me first answer this question: "Are the foods that support female fertility good for increasing men's sperm quality?" The answer to this question is both yes and no. Yes, certain foods that affect women's fertility will affect men positively, while some will not, mainly because the needs of a female's body are different from those of a male's body. Then, how should your spouse eat during this process? I will discuss this subject in my third book, in which I will focus on male fertility. However, I would like to talk about it briefly so that you get an idea of it.

A man's fertility system consists of four parts, namely testicles, the canal system, accessory glands, and penis. Testicles are the part where sperm production happens, and about thirty million sperm are produced every single day under normal circumstances. Assistive ducts carry the sperm that was produced in the testes to the penis. Accessory glands produce the secretion called seminal fluid that feeds sperm and eases their mobility. The penis enables the fertilization of the egg during sexual intercourse. To reproduce, men need a normal amount of adequate and mobile sperm produced by the testes, no blockages in the reproductive system, and no diseases in the reproductive organs.

Male infertility can be related to hormones, genetic causes, kin marriages, varicocele [9], past surgeries, environmental and chemical factors, birth anomalies, and drug use. Just as with menopause in women, a hormonal decline takes place in men after a certain age, and this causes a downgrade in sexual functions.

Men who plan to become fathers:

- Should primarily consult a doctor for a checkup and get treated if there is a hormonal disorder. Celiac disease, cystic fibrosis, chromosomal abnormalities, and canal defects create antibodies that attack sperm.
- Should stop using alcohol, doing drugs, or smoking. Cocaine, marijuana and other similar substances decrease sperm quantity.
- Should, if overweight, lose belly fat; excessive weight impacts male fertility.
- Should not, unless absolutely necessary, use chemical drugs, which reduce sperm quality. X-rays can also impair sperm quality.
- Should exercise regularly.

---

[9] **Varicocele:** a kind of varicosis or abnormal enlargement that forms in the veins returning to the heart from testicles (the sperm-producing sex organs).

- Should get rid of toxins by certain methods such as detoxing or cupping. He should endeavor to cleanse heavy metals from his body.
- Should stay positive.
- Should avoid muscle-strengthening anabolic steroids [10] used for body-building, which shrink ovaries in women and decrease sperm count in men.
- Must implement the proper nutrition program with his spouse.
- Should not wear tight pants or tight underwear. Tight-fitting underwear affects the temperature of the testes and interferes with blood flow. Intensive heat also decreases sperm production and quality.
- Should avoid sitting for long hours while working at a desk or in a cubicle.
- Should refrain from caffeinated and diet beverages and artificial sweeteners like aspartame.

Foods that support male fertility

Being a good father may start long before you think about providing your child with an education at a good school or spending time with him. One of the most important things a father can do for his child is to ensure he contributes the highest possible quality of sperm before the baby is conceived. By doing so, a prospective father will contribute to his child's health positively for a lifetime.

---

[10] **Anabolic steroid:** Drugs that imitate the effects of testosterone or dihydrotestosterone (basic male hormones); the latter is a more powerful form of the first.

Banana, broccoli, strawberry, citrus fruits and their juices; legumes such as lentils and haricot beans; vegetables such as asparagus, avocado, peas, spinach, green beans; and animal foods such as liver, eggs, tuna and yoghurt are necessary for high-quality sperm production. Fat-soluble vitamins A, D, E and K are present in the fatty parts of the food; in other words, if you follow a diet that is very low in fat, it will be hard for you to obtain these significant vitamins in sufficient amounts.

A high vitamin D level in the blood is quite beneficial for women undergoing infertility treatment. Healthy fats are present in olive oil, coconut oil, avocado and hazelnuts, and especially in sunflower seeds and almonds that are rich in vitamin E.

Many studies reveal that tomatoes support male fertility and sperm motility due to their antioxidant lycopene content. You should add a little bit of olive oil on tomatoes to get more of the lycopene. You can cook tomatoes or mash them as well. Moreover:

- Walnuts are quite rich in terms of Omega3 fatty acids and consequently enable sperm vitality and mobility. Eating a handful of walnuts a day will help you manage your blood sugar level as well as serve as a good aphrodisiac.

- Pumpkin seeds provide our body with zinc, which supports sperm development and testosterone production.

- Lentils zfd rich in folate, which is natural folic acid. At the same time, they're a good source of protein and fiber.

- Blueberries shine with their anti-inflammatory features. If you cannot easily eat them, you may mix them into your yoghurt or consume them together with a handful of walnuts.

- Pomegranate is also an excellent fruit that increases blood circulation, reduces the risk of cardiovascular disease and inflammation in the body, and increases sperm quality and sexual desire.

- Bitter chocolate is also among the food items that increase sperm quantity and motility.

Beta carotene

Benefits: This critical phytonutrient helps to regulate hormones and possibly prevent early miscarriages after conception.

Sources: Carrot, melon, pumpkin, sweet potato, spinach, broccoli, cabbage.

B group vitamins

Benefits: All B group vitamins support ovulation. B6 in particular increases the progesterone level necessary to sustain a pregnancy.

Sources: Chickpeas, whole-wheat grains, green-leafy vegetables, meat and eggs.

Bromelain

Benefits: These enzymes primarily digest proteins in the body and help with the implantation of a fertilized egg. In this regard, sufficient intake is important after ovulation.

Sources: Available only in pineapple.

Vitamin C

Benefits: This immunity-increasing vitamin encourages iron absorption and progesterone production. Vitamin C increases fertility in women who suffer from luteal phase defect, which is characterized by insufficient progesterone. It helps to increase sperm health and motility.

Sources: Citrus fruits, mangoes, tomatoes, strawberries, cherries, peas and potatoes.

Choline

Benefits: This water-soluble nutrient is wonderful for the brain health of the mother and the baby. It reduces the rate of babies born with disabilities.

Sources: Egg yolk and cauliflower.

Coenzyme Q10 (CoQ10)

Benefits: This natural enzyme is a superstar supplement for coronary health. It can prevent the decline of egg and sperm quality due to age, as indicated by studies conducted on animals.

Sources: Fish and organ meats such as heart and kidney, and wheat germ.

Vitamin D

Benefits: Vitamin D is fat-soluble. It is vital for the regular production of sex hormones. Research indicates that infertile women generally have low levels of vitamin D. According to a study conducted by Yale School of Medicine, vitamin D is low in the majority of women. While vitamin D improves general fertility, it also reduces inflammation in the body.

Sources: Sun, salmon, mackerel, tuna fish, dairy products with high fat.

Vitamin E

Benefits: Specialists state that the liquid surrounding the egg is important for its development. This liquid contains a considerable amount of vitamin E, which improves the health of the sperm. Vitamin E has also antioxidant features for both sexes.

Sources: Avocado, wheat germ oil, sweet potatoes, green-leafy vegetables, whole-grain cereals, almonds, peanuts and hazelnuts.

Folic acid

Benefits: Folic acid is the synthetic folate form of B group vitamins known as B9. Folic acid enables proper neural tube development in the baby's brain and spinal cord. It is very important for women trying to conceive, therefore folic acid pills are generally prescribed by doctors. Women in the USA typically use supplements, as they do not get enough folate from their diet. Getting daily folic acid supplements of 400 mcg (micrograms) is important for getting pregnant. Folic acid also increases men's sperm count. In a study carried out at the University of California at Berkeley, a 20% increase was observed in the sperm count of men who were taking folic acid.

Sources: Beans, orange juice, green-leafy vegetables and fortified grains.

Iron

Benefits: Pregnancy usually causes women to become anemic. If a woman has low iron levels during pre-pregnancy, she is likely to have ovulation problems.

Sources: Meat, egg, fish, beans, broccoli, spinach and whole-grain cereals.

Omega3 fatty acids

Benefits: The human body cannot produce these naturally. Omega3 fatty acids increase blood flow to the uterus, enable the release of the egg, and balance hormones. Preliminary studies reveal that it can also help with fetal brain development and IQ level.

Sources: Flaxseed, flaxseed oil, salmon, mackerel, codfish, sardines, anchovy, herring and walnuts.

Selenium

Benefits: It increases sperm motility in men and estrogen in women.

Sources: Peas, hazelnuts, green-leafy vegetables, whole-grain cereals and fish.

Zinc

Benefits: Zinc helps to increase sperm motility and its general quality. It is also important for female reproductive health. The U.S. Centers for Disease Control and Prevention linked early miscarriages are linked to low levels of zinc.

Sources: Oysters, fish, meat, egg, poultry, wheat germ and pumpkin seed.

Other ways to increase male fertility

According to research by the American Society for Reproductive Medicine, men who consume more fruits and vegetables have higher fertility. When researchers compared the diets of two groups of men who were able and unable to help their partners conceive within a year, results showed that 83% of the infertile men had a low intake of fruits and vegetables, defined as fewer than five servings a day, compared with 40% of the fertile men. The research indicated that men who eat little amounts of fruits and vegetables have the lowest sperm motility.

Md. Vivian Lewis, Professor of Obstetrics & Gynecology at Rochester University, says sperm quality is affected by dietary antioxidant intake. Antioxidants contained in fruits and vegetables help to prevent damage to sperm. Lewis states that glutathione and kryptoxanthin antioxidants, which are especially abundant in fibrous greens, tomatoes, peppers, and oranges, are related to vigorous and healthy sperm.

Let's talk about the much-debated relationship between technology and health. There are various studies and opinions about technology's effect on male infertility in the U.S. Some researchers have linked weak sperm to mobile phone use and recommend that men preparing for fatherhood should reduce the time spent using one. A study of 361 men within the framework of infertility found that those who spent a lot of time on their mobile devices daily were more likely to have unhealthy sperm. Men who spent over four hours on their mobiles daily had a lower sperm count, lower sperm motility, and a higher number of sperm with abnormal morphology than those who did not use a mobile device at all. The difference between these two groups varied between 30% and 50%.

Ashok Agarwal, the andrology director of the Ohio Cleveland Clinic Glickman Urological and Kidney Institute, also says electromagnetic waves spread by mobile devices can potentially weaken sperm.

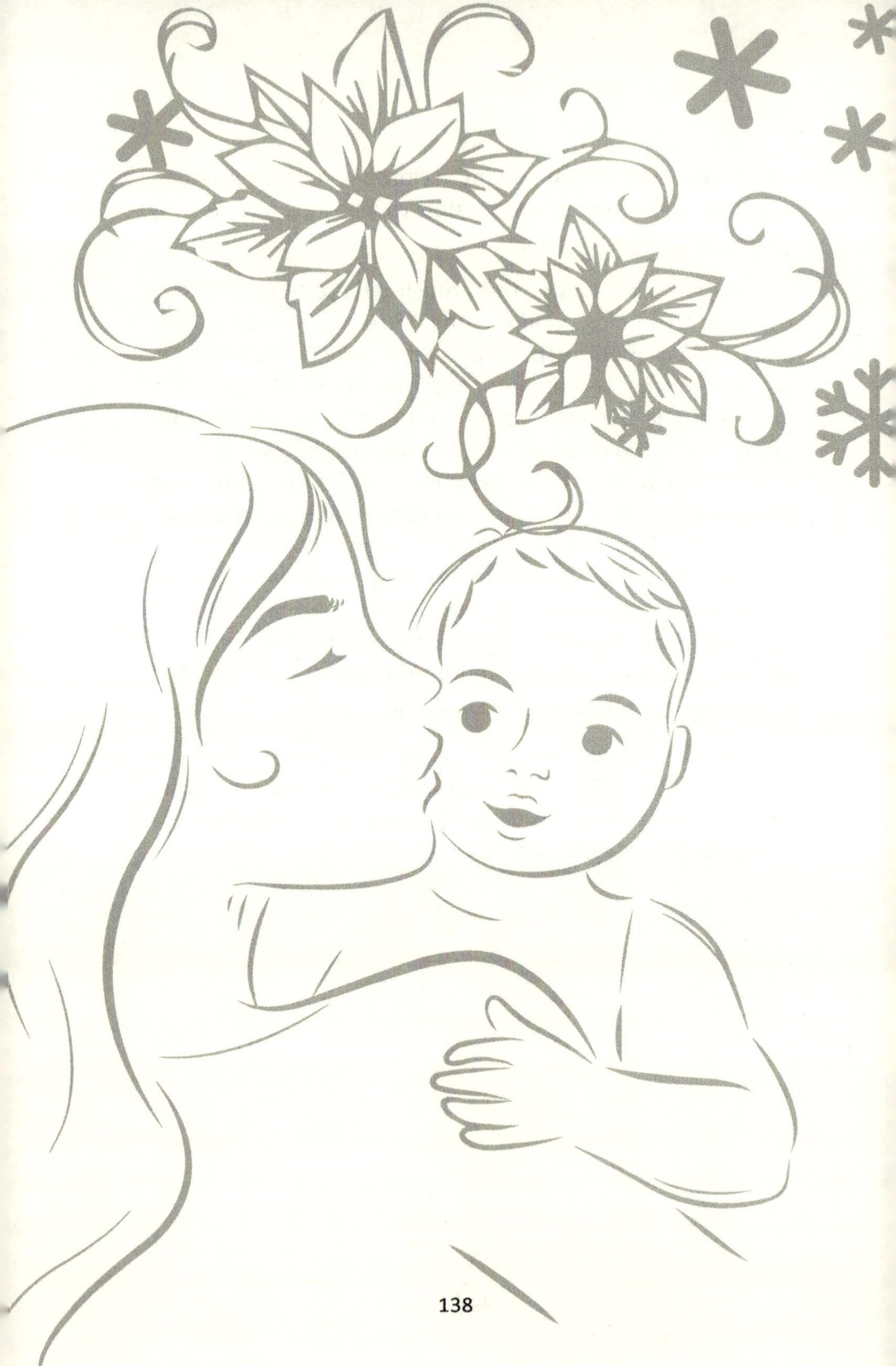

Chapter Five

DISEASES AND NUTRITION

Every country cope with a high rate of certain diseases that originate from its living conditions. In this sense, the most common diseases observed in Turkey are diabetes, high blood pressure, heart and cardiovascular diseases, cancer, shortness of breath, calcification, hernia-sciatica and ulcer-gastritis. The two major causes underlying these diseases are unhealthy diet and lack of exercise.

Thyroid Hormone and Fertility

In recent years, we've seen an increase in health issues stemming from thyroid hormone problems. Many women take thyroid pills to keep their hormones at desired levels. Thyroid hormones continuously interact with estrogen and progesterone to sustain the function of the ovaries and enable the maturation of an egg. Pregnancy is affected negatively in all cases when the thyroid is toxicant, lazy or overactive.

I recommend that any woman who experiences symptoms such as fatigue, lack of sleep, weight problems, mood changes, intestinal problems, muscle and joint problems, problematic menstrual cycles, hair loss, skin issues, heart rate and blood pressure issues, throat enlargement or eyelid retraction, should consult an endocrinologist. A family history of thyroid disease is also important.

Women with hypothyroid problems should focus on getting enough healthy proteins, fats, whole-grain cereals, colorful fruits and vegetables, and anti-inflammatory foods. Seaweed, seafood, organic milk, eggs and strawberry support our body's iodine needs. You can get selenium from organic fat-free meat, hazelnuts, cheese, eggs, liver, butter, cold-water fish, onion, garlic, leeks, mushrooms, tomatoes and green vegetables. Foods that will supply you with zinc are cheese, duck, goose, turkey, herring, peanuts, pumpkin seeds, whole-grain cereals, cucumbers, watermelon skin, peas, carrots, and beets. As for l-tyrosine, used in the synthesis of thyroid hormone, you need to consume beans, sesame, pumpkin seeds, and organic chicken if available. You should eat cold-water fish for Omega3. Vitamins E, C, A and B are other vitamins your body needs. If you have hypothyroid issues, avoid eating excessively, consuming wheat gluten, inflammatory foods (such as processed fats, sugar, flour and alcohol), excessive salt and soy. Also, keep away from flaxseed or vegetables like cabbage, which pose a risk of inhibited thyroid function.

Thyroid hormones affect all cells in the body. For this reason, the entire body is affected when there is a thyroid dysfunction.

Diabetes Is there a link between diabetes and fertility? In the U.S., type 2 diabetes has been investigated in cases of unexplained infertility. According to the American Diabetes Association, even though there is no direct link between diabetes and fertility, some women who are suffering from diabetes but can get pregnant may have problems in sustaining the pregnancy. A high glucose level raises the miscarriage risk by 30% to 60%.

It is a common view that diabetes emerges more often in pregnancy. Babies born to mothers who experience gestational diabetes mellitus (GDM) during pregnancy are usually overweight, and the chance of being diagnosed with diabetes is higher for these women in future years.

Cells use the glucose they need by means of the insulin hormone produced in the pancreas. If the body does not produce insulin, this is called type 1 diabetes. Type 2 diabetes, on the other hand, appears when an insufficient amount of insulin is produced or the cells in the body do not react properly to insulin. It is estimated that there are over seven million diabetes patients in Turkey, a number projected to rise to ten million in the near future. In some cases, almost a decade can pass between the onset of the disease and its advanced stages. You can find out whether you have diabetes by taking a simple blood test.

If we lend an ear to the Turkish Diabetes Foundation, we can learn about ways to avoid this disease. These include having plenty of whole grains and fibrous foods on your dining table, consuming fish twice a week, consuming more fresh vegetables and fruits, limiting sugar and salt to the daily needs of our body, drinking lots of water, and taking at least 5,000 steps a day.

If a risk for diabetes exists, doctors recommend that such women who are trying to conceive keep their daily sugar levels under control. As a matter of fact, this is necessary for any woman who would like to support her fertility!

Hypertension and Heart Disease

Hypertension or high blood pressure is a chronic health problem and can cause many complications. However, it's difficult to assert any direct effect on fertility. It does not affect ovulation or the embryo, but it may affect implantation, which is the embedding of the embryo in the uterus. If a prospective mother experiencing high blood pressure would like to have a smooth pregnancy, she should drink lots of water and definitely keep away from salt. Salt consumption can lead to pre-eclampsia, a complication that can be defined as toxemia of pregnancy after the sixth month.

Women are luckier in terms of cardio health, because estrogen has a diminishing effect on arteriosclerosis. Coronary arteriosclerosis, coronary embolism and heart attack complications are rarely observed in women during peak times of fertility, when estrogen hormone is high. For this reason, heart problems typically arise after menopause in women.

Polycystic Ovary Syndrome

Polycystic ovary syndrome (PCOS) occurs when many small benign cysts develop in the ovaries, and it is generally observed in women under 35 years of age. This syndrome stems from abnormal LH and FSH secretions by the pituitary gland. PCOS causes irregular ovulation, sometimes rare menstrual bleeding, such as once or twice a year, and a rise of androgens (male hormones). Androgens transform fat tissue into estrogen, and estrogen increases LH production. As a result, a vicious cycle emerges. This vicious cycle can be broken with weight loss or suppression of the ovaries.

In cases of polycystic ovary syndrome, absence of, or rare, occurrence of ovulation prevents pregnancy. Medications that stimulate ovulation are required under such circumstances. Weight loss and medication treatment usually yield nice results and pregnancy happens by itself.

Allergy and Fertility

Many couples are unaware of the fact that their lifestyle habits affect their fertility. Factors like taking hot baths on a regular basis and consuming coffee or fast food take a toll on fertility. What if certain foods that are healthy for the majority are not healthy for some? For example, people suffering from allergies and intolerance issues.

The most commonly observed intolerance is celiac disease, in which the small intestine has a lifelong sensitivity to gluten. Gluten is a complex protein that is present in grains such as wheat, barley and rye. All of us are often exposed to it. Gluten creates problems by affecting the absorption of natural food by the intestines and impairing the immune system. Improper nutrition also harms the reproductive system over time, as organ systems in our body depend on nutrition. Gluten can cause irregular menstrual cycles and even infertility in due course.

It decreases sperm quality and quantity in men. People suffering from such an intolerance should support their fertility by following a gluten-free diet. You may have gluten intolerance if you continuously feel bloated and gassy in the abdomen; if you have constipation, diarrhea, irritable bowel, joint and bone aches, canker sores in the mouth, itchy rashes; if you are moody or depressed.

Another intolerance we frequently see is yeast intolerance. Yeast is present in many products like fermented drinks, bread, cheese, vinegar, preserves, ketchup, mayonnaise and bouillon. If you experience bloating, dizziness, fatigue, watery eyes, heartburn, nausea, or skin rashes, or have to deal with sneezing and a stuffy nose whenever you consume a yeasted product, chances are you have yeast allergy.

Although no evidence suggests that milk intolerance affects fertility, some doctors have found that pregnancy happens more easily when milk is excluded from the diet of people who are sensitive to casein and lactose. This is something we might want to keep in mind.

THE MOST COMMON MYTHS ABOUT FERTILITY

Md. Angeline Beltsos, of the Chicago Vios Fertility Institute, says that millions of couples spend years trying to prevent pregnancy, and for this reason may face problems when they decide to have a baby. Infertility can happen to anyone, and many prospective parents do not understand the factors that affect their individual fertility potential, regardless of their age, ethnicity, intelligence, intellectual capacity or diligence. According to Md. Angeline Beltsos, the following are some of the most common myths she hears from patients.

1. "He does not have a fertility problem; he is already a dad."

Contrary to popular belief, male fertility is limited. Just as with women, the fertility of men also decreases with age, especially after the age of 40. Researchers point to a direct link between the age of fatherhood and increased risk of autism and schizophrenia. The genetic mutation men go through is fourfold that in women. The older a man gets, the lower the volume of mobile and healthy semen becomes.

2. "The women in my family had babies in their 40s, so I should be fine."

Even though family history is taken into account during treatment, it neither supports nor prevents fertility potential. Previous successful pregnancies may not guarantee a good route for future pregnancies. According to the U.S. Centers for Disease Control and Prevention, 11% of couples with a single child experience secondary infertility within a year. While the chance of pregnancy is 20% for a woman who is 30 years old, this rate goes down by 5% when the woman turns 40.

3. "I smoke, so I'll have to quit when I get pregnant."

The American Association of Reproductive Health estimates that as much as 13% of female infertility diagnoses stem from smoking. Believe it or not, smoking about five cigarettes a day is linked to low fertility rates in both men and women.

4. "We are having sex 24 hours after the ovulation."

It is not possible to fall pregnant after ovulation ends. Ovulation happens once a month, when the egg is released into the fallopian tubes, roughly 7–10 days prior to the menstrual cycle of a woman. The sperm must find an egg within this period in one or two days for the pregnancy to take place.

To increase the chance of success, have sex right before and during ovulation, as sperm can survive in the reproductive tract for three days. Women with irregular menstrual cycles should see a specialist to identify their ovulation time. Ovulatory disorders are most commonly observed fertility diagnoses in women.

5. "I don't have to worry about my eggs until the age of 40."

Although a baby girl is born with seven million eggs, this number drops to four hundred thousand around the time of puberty. A woman produces about 400–500 eggs throughout her life, and her ovarian reserve declines as she gets older. A woman's egg supply starts declining at the end of her 20s but decreases rapidly after the age of 35.

6. "I exercise and do yoga. I am perfectly fit. My age shouldn't affect my fertility."

Healthy body and mind can increase fertility but cannot reverse the age of ovaries and sperm. Age is a critical component of fertility for both sexes.

7. "We can lose weight together but..."

When men or women lose extra weight, hormonal changes that can affect ovulation and sperm production take place in the body. The good news is, when couples lose weight together, this serves as an opportunity for them to become more active and increase their fertility by forming a team. It's estimated that 70% of infertile women are obese but losing 5%–10% of body weight can increase fertility in both sexes.

8. "Only women need to use supplements before pregnancy."

It has been known for a long time that women need to take folic acid to prevent certain birth defects. However, folic acid is currently accepted as an important supplement for men to increase fertility. Researchers at University of California Berkeley discovered that men with low folic acid in their diet have higher chromosomal abnormalities in their sperm. Coenzyme Q10 increases sperm count and motility, and vitamin E improves low sperm count.

9. "Sexually transmitted diseases affect my health, but not my conception efforts."

STDs can affect the ability to produce a baby in both men and women. Such diseases can cause blockages and lesions in male reproductive organs. When left untreated in women, they can cause pelvic inflammatory disease, which is one of the leading causes of infertility.

10. "We are having sex every day in order to conceive."

According to a research published in New England Journal of Medicine, chances of conception increase only very slightly when having sex daily and having sex every other day are compared. If a man has a normal sperm count, his sperm concentration diminishes in the case of daily sex.

Chapter Six

FREQUENTLY ASKED QUESTIONS

Will a wrong diet prevent me from getting pregnant?

A wrong diet means malnutrition. In the case of malnutrition, your hormonal balance can go awry. As egg and sperm health are directly linked to nutrition, your current nutrition will affect your pregnancy and even your baby's health.

What is the effect of body weight on fertility?

A person who does not otherwise have an infertility problem might not have a baby simply because s/he is overweight. This is true not only for women but also for men. It has been identified that the probability of conception declines by 8% in significantly overweight women and 18% in obese women. At the same time, 12% of couples suffering from infertility are observed to experience this problem due to weight issues. Even though this percentage also includes underweight couples, the majority are overweight. Excessive weight can cause infertility for both sexes by creating a hormonal imbalance.

I do not seem overweight, but my body fat percentage is high. How will this affect me when it comes to conceiving?

Your body fat rate is important in terms of fertility. Sex hormones dissolve in fat; for this reason, the fat rate and sex hormones are highly related in our body. High body fat can create irregularity in estrogen production and menstrual cycles. As for men, excessive weight causes fat accumulation and a subsequent higher temperature around testes; this in turn causes a decline in sperm quantity and quality.

The total body fat percentage of a woman should be approximately 20% of her body weight. Estrogen and other hormones that are necessary for ovulation cannot be produced regularly in women who are very thin and have a body fat rate lower than 20%. Having a higher fat rate translates into overproduction of these hormones, and this also leads to irregular ovulation.

One thing you should keep in mind is that undergoing an unhealthy diet to lose weight in hopes of getting pregnant will also affect your fertility adversely. You should lose weight by means of a healthy diet and routine exercise instead of ruining your hormone levels with shock diets or staying hungry for long periods of time.

How do tea, herbal teas and coffee affect fertility? Which is good, which is harmful?

We know that caffeine increases stress and anxiety levels and decreases blood flow to uterus. At the same time, coffee increases the risk of miscarriage, creates a hormonal imbalance, decreases sperm quality, elevates the body's acidity and lowers calcium levels. Even if you cannot give it up completely, you need to lower your daily consumption to minimum. Tea is a better alternative, but you should also consume it in moderation. Herbal teas should not be consumed a lot unless you are sure of their content and safety. It is critically important to consume right amounts of herbs which are known to improve hormonal balance!

How shall we calculate daily calorie intake or glycemic load?

Glycemic load is more important. We should endeavor to kep our hormone levels balanced by consuming carbohydrates with a low glycemic index to prevent rapid fluctuations in our blood sugar. For example, the glycemic indexes of white rice, brown rice and bulgur are 64, 55 and 46 respectively. So, we should prefer bulgur out of the three.

There are different perspectives on counting calories. It's better to pay attention to proper nutrition instead of worrying about calories.

Will detox contribute to fertility?

Getting ready for pregnancy by purifying your body of accumulated toxins will absolutely contribute to your fertility. A large portion of toxins accumulate in the liver, kidneys and fat cells. As the body benefits from fat cells to a huge extent during pregnancy and nursing, toxins can be directly transmitted to the baby. Detoxing prior to pregnancy will be beneficial to prevent this occurrence.

Still, cleansing our daily habits and eating habits from toxins may be more effective than doing detoxes that will wear down the body. Short-term cures can be implemented by using herbs that cleanse the liver, kidneys, uterus and the entire system.

Do you support green juice or blending? What is their impact on our health?

Even though green juice is beneficial, it is healthier to consume fruits and vegetables with pulp. Green juices that consist of 20% fruit juice and 80% vegetable juice provide us with more minerals and vitamins than we can normally get by eating. Consuming food in liquid form facilitates absorption. However, when we extract their juice, we lose the fiber that we need. Smoothies contain fiber, but their digestion is not as easy as that of green juice. Green juice is healthier than fruit juice. You can consume many healthy vegetables by using different recipes to turn them into green juice. Carrot, beet, celery, parsley, cucumber, green apple and pear are some examples. You can also add flax seed or chia seed to these. Keep in mind that you need to use these in a balanced way within your diet to rest your stomach and body. You can choose green juices or smoothies when you want to have a light dinner.

Do you recommend food items such as tofu, krill oil, chia seed, flax seed, spiranula or any special foods to enhance fertility?

One should be careful about the tofu produced from soya. Soya affects the tissues by changing estrogen and testosterone production, concentration, metabolization, and elimination from the body. Soya which contains herbal estrogens and environments with high estrogen concentration can hinder hormonal influences. If it is in an environment with low estrogen concentration, it can increase the influence of estrogen. Phytoestrogens act in a way that is similar to estrogen, but they also react to estrogen. In other words, if there is excessive estrogen in the body, they remove the excessive effect of estrogen by getting linked to estrogen receptors, or they act like estrogen if there is little estrogen in the body. The two most common groups of phytoestrogens are isoflavones and lignans. Isoflavones are present in soy beans, haricot beans, lentils, peas, vegetables and tea. Lignans are present in all grains, flax seed, sesame, sunflower seed, peanuts, olives, cherries, peaches, plums, apples, pears, carrots, broccolis, onion, garlic, fennel, raspberries, and hops. Phytoestrogens are very strong antioxidants. Women who consume soy get positive results from infertility treatments.

How can we use technology for fertility?

Even though there are many apps available to help you track ovulation and menstruation, there are barely any for fertility enhancement. A few mobile apps are available at Apple Store and Google Play. The "How to Boost Fertility: Pregnancy" mobile application helps users improve their fertility with things they do on their own. Here, you can get news about recent research on fertility, a list of good and harmful foods, and suggestions for solving lifestyle-related issues. "Get Pregnant-Fertility Self-Treat" is a source that focuses on massage. You can learn to do easy massages on certain areas by watching videos that feature methods applied in China. The "Barbados Fertility App," developed by a fertility clinic, contains a great deal of information about ovulation, a fertility calendar, information on IVF methods, and FAQs answered by specialists are included in this application.

Do you recommend light, diet and diabetic products?

I do not recommend light products unless these products need to be used due to a diabetes issue. Regular milk contains 3% fat, 5% carbohydrates, 3% proteins. While there is an average of 2% fat in light milk, its carbohydrate rate or glycemic index is high. This is not something we prefer in the Motherhood Diet.

What is the relationship between sleep and fertility?

Healthy sleep affects fertility directly. The body repairs and cleanses itself as well as regulating hormones and chemical balance during sleep. Irregular sleep causes weight gain and hormonal imbalance by slowing down the metabolism. As a result, healthy production of estrogen, progesterone, LH and FSH are related to healthy sleep. If sleep irregularity is chronic, the leptin hormone, which affects ovulation, is also impacted negatively. A study conducted on night-shift nurses in 2012 showed that irregular sleep patterns may lead to menstruation irregularities and breech birth by affecting physical rhythm. In the same way, irregular sleep increases the secretion of cortisol and adrenocorticotrophic (ACTH) hormones, both of which are known to affect fertility negatively in females and males.

Women with irregular sleep patterns have low body temperature. This, in turn, renders it more difficult to identify the fertility window based on body temperature. Women are recommended to get eight hours of sleep per day.

Do digestive disorders such as constipation affect fertility?

The important thing is to find the source of disorders. In other words, constipation should be further noted if it happens due to fibroid tumors; similarly, symptoms such as heartburn and diarrhea may originate from reproductive disorders like endometriosis. Digestive system disorders also indicate whether you are eating healthfully and exercising correctly. If you are experiencing any health issues in your digestive system, you must be doing something wrong, and you need to interfere with the process by finding the source.

Is it possible to get pregnant during menopause? If yes, which extra nutrients do I need?

Menopause is a process that has three phases. In the perimenopause phase, which lasts two to eight years, irregular periods and changes in hormonal levels are observed. It is possible to fall pregnant and give birth to healthy babies during this period. In the second phase, which starts with the cessation of the menstrual period, hormonal changes become more rapid. The third stage, which we call post-menopause, lasts until the completion of hormonal changes around the ages of 58 to 60. The chance of healthy pregnancy and birth after the age of 40 is high in women who protect their ovarian, uterine and hormonal health.

Does the use of artificial sweeteners affect fertility?

FDA (American Food and Drug Administration) states that sweeteners, except for saccharin and stevia, can be used during pregnancy in small quantities. However, natural nutritionists think that these products are toxic and should definitely not be used.

There are some rumors that stevia is used as a traditional contraceptive in South America, but research indicates that it does not yield such an effect when used in normal doses. Studies continue regarding this matter. There is much debate about aspartame. In his experiments carried out on animals, Md. Madelon Price observed that aspartame paves the way for infertility by preventing prolactin secretion. Changing your behavioral habits and making your body get used to sugar-free instead of consuming foods and beverages that contain artificial sweeteners is considered the best option.

Is raw meat or raw fish consumption harmful?

Food such as salami, hotdogs, pepperoni, pastrami, steak tartar a la turca, and carpaccio are prepared without cooking. Even though they go through a process, this does not destroy all the bacteria in these products. It will be beneficial to avoid such food during a period in which you would like to increase your fertility.

How does a raw vegetable and fruit diet affect fertility?

The most important thing for the followers of a raw food diet should be getting vitamins, minerals, fats and proteins in sufficient amounts, just like vegans and vegetarians. Food items lose some of their nutritional value depending on the way of cooking. You may consume raw food as part of your diet, but if you are eating only raw food, you need to go out in the sun and enable your body to produce vitamin D, consume plenty of green-leafy vegetables to get vitamin B, and obtain necessary fat from products such as avocado, coconut, dried nuts, sesame and olives.

Are preserved food and pickles good or harmful for me?

Food with high salt content affects fertility negatively. If you are buying preserves or preserved products instead of making them at home, there might be various chemicals in their packaging which may lead to infertility.

Polyamines are organic compounds that play a key role in cell growth. Although their exact function is still not known, it has been observed that cell growth is seriously prevented in case of their absence.

Fertility specialists at the Sydney Fertility Clinic studied the dietary impacts and confirmed the effects of polyamines on female fertility. Researchers observed that polyamines that arose during pregnancy were important in terms of healthy development of DNA in an embryo. According to Md. David Knight, the absence of polyamines can lead to infertility in women. Studies conducted on old mice show that normal pregnancy rates tripled within two months after the mice were given polyamine compounds. Even though findings are not very scientific at this point, results are encouraging. Polyamines, putrescine, spermidine and spermine components are being specially tested at the time in terms of their effects on pregnancy.

Nutritional sources of polyamine components are the products that we can easily find and consume in daily life.

Putrescine: Aged cheeses such as kashar, roquefort, and tulum, potatoes, preserved frozen vegetables, orange and frozen shrimp.

Spermidine: Aged cheeses, soybean, processed tea, vegetable, potatoes and fresh bread.

Spermine: Grains, preserved or frozen vegetables, meat products, red meat and poultry.

Should I avoid stale products?

Consuming fresh food is safer than eating food that was prepared a while ago. Mold can grow in products that has been waiting. Mold is a form of fungi and produces mycotoxin that affects our health adversely. Mold is not always visible; therefore, I suggest you opt for fresh products as it is impossible to know whether the molding process has started.

Will implementing a ketogenic diet increase the chance of pregnancy?

A study conducted in 2012 revealed that ketogenic diet (a type of diet concentrating on fat and protein) hindered brain and physical development in babies of pregnant women who followed such a diet. Diets that are made without consuming any carbohydrates cannot provide us with balanced nutrition. We need to include slow carbohydrates in our diets rather than consuming zero carbohydrates.

http://bmcpregnancychildbirth.biomedcentral.com/articles/10.1186/1471-2393-13-198

How does an alkaline diet affect fertility?

It is beneficial to consume alkaline food that will help to reduce the acid surplus in the body. Most fruits, vegetables and nuts help with alkaline production. It will be sufficient to keep away from products that increase acid production, such as caffeine, alcohol, sugar and tobacco. If you look at the food range, you will see that harmful food is acidic while healthy food such as vegetables and fruits are alkaline.

SOURCES:

http://www.ted.com/talks/kelly_mcgonigal_how_to_make_stress_your_friend/transcript?language=en#t-374725

http://www.ted.com/talks/tyrone_hayes_penelope_jagessar_chaffer_the_toxic_baby/transcript?language=en#t-4083

Lewis, Sally. 50 Things You Can Do Today to Increase Your Fertility, West Sussex: Summersdale Publications, 2011. Ve http://www.zestnaturalhealth.co.nz/preconception-care-and-fertility/how-effective-is-preconceptive-care/)

TURKİYE'YE OZGU BESİN VE BESLENME REHBERİ (NUTRIENT & NUTRITION GUIDE PECULIAR TO TURKEY) Ankara 2015 Hacettepe University Prof. Md. Halit Tanju Besler, Prof. Md. Neslisah Rakicioglu, Assoc. Prof. Aylin Ayaz, Assoc. Prof. Zehra Buyuktuncer Demirel, Assoc. Prof. Hulya Gokmen Ozel, Assoc. Prof. Gulhan Eroglu Samur, Assoc. Prof. Emine Akal Yildiz, Assistant Assoc. Prof. Pelin Bilgic, Assistant Assoc. Prof. Derya Dikmen, Assistant Assoc. Prof. Zeynep Goktas, Assistant Assoc. Prof. Mevlude Kizil, Assistant Assoc. Prof. Asli Akyol Mutlu, Assistant Assoc. Prof. Reyhan Nergiz Unal, Md. Mehmet Fisunoglu, Md. Atila Gulec, Research Assistant Seda Ciftci, Specialist Research Assistant Gozde Ede, Specialist Research Assistant Ruveyda Esra Ercim, Specialist Research Assistant Arzu Kabasakal, Specialist Research Assistant Damla Yilmaz, Specialist Research Assistant Armagan Yuruk

www.sciencedaily.com/releases/2008/01/080121080402.htm

http://natural-fertility-info.com/hypothyroidism-reproductive-health.html

http://www.thebump.com/a/hypertension-getting-pregnant

http://www.usenature.com/articles/nutrition/254-allergies-and-infertility#.V-z9L_CLTIU

Made in the USA
Coppell, TX
04 November 2026

11282135R00100